HARD!

Maintaining Potency, Eliminating Erectile Dysfunction, And Enjoying Healthy Sex for Life

Robin D. Ader

© 2014 Copyright Robin D. Ader
1st edition © 2011 Robin D. Ader
2nd edition © 2012 Robin D. Ader

Hundredth Shire Publishing, LLC
http://HShirePublishing.com

ISBN-13: 978-0-9895435-4-5
ISBN-10: 0989543544

Table of Contents

Disclaimer:

These are my thoughts, my experiences, and what I did to get over my dysfunction. I share it with you because I believe that if it worked for me it should work for most guys; I took no extraordinary measures, engaged in no costly therapies, and performed no activity that any ambulatory guy can't match.

However, nothing I have written here has been confirmed and proven scientifically using large, statistically significant numbers of men tested under the scrutiny of controlled circumstances and professional observation. It's just me. Nothing I suggest has been investigated, endorsed, or underwritten by the FDA, which, by the way, has approved any number of drugs that have subsequently been removed from the market after people died from them.

My hypothesis has not been reviewed by any medical authority.

All I can tell you is that it worked for me. Give it a try at your own risk—or reward. I found a solution. These thoughts may help you find yours, too.

But it is not my intention to provide you with the ability to diagnose yourself. Be sure you seek medical attention if you can't perform sexually, as it may be a symptom of a greater issue. In Chapter 4, *Dead Men Don't Get Laid*, I relate my experience getting a full medical examination. Pay special attention to the section entitled, "See your doctor anyway."

And finally, I find it clumsy to replace the word "woman" with "partner" in every instance. What I've written is a reflection on my personal experience, from the perspective of a heterosexual man with a female partner. There is no doubt that ED can impact gay relationships—perhaps doubly—so I cannot fathom why everything I say here wouldn't apply to gay men; it's just the pronouns that differ. Occasionally, however, I refer to that vagina thing; ignore those passages.

x

Preface to the Third Edition

Half full or half empty? The two previous versions of HARD! took aim primarily at eliminating Erectile Dysfunction. With this edition, I'm focusing on Erection *Function*.

Ample space is given to the causes of dysfunction, but new sections have been added highlighting those things we can do, foods we can eat, and mental exercises we can perform to improve function once dysfunction has been overcome. In this way, this guide can take you the full voyage from disappointment to wild approval.

In the intervening two years since the second edition, I've found a mate, eleven years my junior, with whom I'll likely go the distance, dying in each other's arms exhausted not just from a round of explosive sex, but having used up all the orgasms we're allowed in a lifetime. With this lady, I get [almost] a daily status-check of whether what I'm doing is working as well as we'd both hope. So, I've added a section discussing those things that can kill an erection for a night, soften one's potency for a short time, or shut you down completely, faster than you can imagine.

And I offer an opportunity in this edition, the ***One-Week Challenge*** that could restore your erectile function all by itself. Your participation and feedback are encouraged.

Forward

This book is rated "R"

This is *not* a clinical, academic, medical treatment of male sexuality. You don't need another respectful discussion that speaks to you as if you're an adolescent in a high school health class.

HARD! is written by a man—for men—in the words, phrases, expressions, and with the irreverence that is common to man-speak. This book uses the language and allusion that is the common currency of men in the hallowed halls of government, the ivory towers of multinational corporations, health club locker rooms, and the local bar.

Most importantly, it's written by a man who's been there and pulled himself back from the abyss.

I'm going to suggest how, regardless of your age, you can maintain the ability to get an erection with the objective of confidently engaging in loving and fun sex when a woman offers her most intimate self to you. The suggestions presented in this book also promote overall well-being, allowing you to participate in healthy and animated congress with that woman—aka—*great sex!*

That's what *HARD!* is all about.

The subject is critical to men who approach or have crossed the half century mark in their lives. It is also increasingly important to younger men among whom erectile dysfunction is growing in frequency as early as their twenties.

Still, it's necessary to take a journey through the body so you may understand the underlying issues, and make educated judgments regarding your lifestyle. I'm teaching you to fish rather than handing you the fish.

And Something for the Ladies, Too

If you, dear lady, seek more meaningful and gratifying sexual experiences with the man or men in your life, then this book will be a valuable resource.

A good portion of the general information and some of the sexual advice that I present is as applicable to your health and satisfaction as it is to a man's.

In addition to the indispensable information presented for men, there is also much from which you can benefit by understanding the sexual function of the guys from whom you demand your pleasures.

Further, as a couple, your cooperation in the dining room, as well as the bedroom, will be essential to the rejuvenation and enhancement of your man's performance.

In this case, ladies, ***payback could be Heaven***.

PART I — Foreplay of Sorts

Chapter 1: A Preview of the Plan

Let's start on the buffet line at the all-you-can-eat barbeque chicken and ribs joint down the road. You are presented with dozens of choices. They all look good, but some are better than others and it's that small difference that makes you take the ribs instead of the chicken, moves you a helping of the bacon and beans, and to leave the cole slaw behind, and gets you to finish with the brownies and ice cream rather than apple pie.

But in addition to leaving the chicken, coleslaw, and pie, you're also leaving your potency at the hot table. It's a choice you've made.

If I said that you have to give up ribs, beans, and ice cream, you'd never buy this book. Hell, the plan never would have worked for me, either. But I'm not saying you have to give up anything, not completely, at least. There are concessions to be made, for sure, because if you change nothing, nothing changes, and your *limpy* will stay just that way.

This is not a diet plan. But what you eat has a lot to do with what's killing your dick, even if you're fairly active and count calories. It's a matter of what your foods do to you on the inside, that isn't necessarily visible on the outside that counts.

What I present is a Cafeteria Plan from which you've got dozens of choices and can still enjoy half of them. Deciding which you'll select is up to you. And among those selections are lifestyle options, not just food choices. I will suggest ways you can cut down or eliminate erection-killing substances from your food, drink, and environment. I provide two physical exercises that take less than twenty minutes of your time when performed ten minutes, twice daily, one of which I designed specifically for erectile health. I will discuss a way of overcoming the psychological factors that can lead to erectile dysfunction.

And then we discuss promoting higher levels of erectile function.

Let me give away the punch line. What's been killing your potency is not any one thing.

Erectile dysfunction is the cumulative effect of everything you do to torture your body and mind.

For many men, the worst offenders—those actions that directly affect your ability to get an erection—will gladly be exchanged for a hard dick, along with the confidence you can perform great and frequent sex.

I provide the knowledge of why these things are harmful. I explain how an erection works, and how each *offender* kills your ability to get hard. This insight will help you to make decisions regarding the future of your sex life.

This book describes an overall health regimen, for what the hell good is a stiff dick, if your delivery mechanism—the rest of your body—can't perform; lung capacity, a strong heart, and body stamina are all essential to making love.

And a note for the single guys: what woman will take you to her bed if you look like shit. You don't have to be slim and ripped, but you can't look like you're near death either.

Chapter 2: My Personal Story

I am a heterosexual man who, through my twenties and thirties, had a prolific sex life. I owned a travel agency, bounced around the world, and had experiences that, if I told you, you'd tell me to my face I was full of bullshit.

The 1970s were pre-HIV and pre-Herpes. Virtually all sexually active women were on birth control pills, and meeting a woman at a bar, and having a few drinks followed by sex, was common. I had acceptably good looks and a personality, so among my contemporaries, I did well. I maintained my bachelor lifestyle through my thirty-ninth birthday.

Then I got married just after I turned forty. This was my first—and to this writing—only marriage.

We were a cliché. We stayed together years longer than we should have for the sake of our daughter in an arrangement devoid of intimacy. We divorced after seventeen years.

Close to the legal end of my marriage, I was fifty-seven, I received a call from an old lover who I hadn't seen in twenty years. Memories of our sex-charged relationship came back in force. I gladly reconnected with her and after a brief re-courtship, we were back in bed.

At the conclusion of our first coital romp, I rolled over and, being the wordsmith that I am, said, "Just like old times." She responded, "Yeah, but with a lot more gasping for air."

I knew I was woefully out of shape and the burning in my lungs confirmed that. Like most guys, I presumed that I would have the stamina to perform "basic" sex.

I had lied; it was not like "old times" or any time in my life, ever. While I ultimately managed to go the distance, much of my exertion was due to... well… going the distance, and not the pleasure of the run. I thought I was out of practice. I thought I was having performance anxiety. But in the morning, the second go-round wasn't any better.

This lady still cared for me, and gave me every benefit of the doubt; she understood that decades had passed since we had been together and we were both more *mature*. While I had not been in the arms or vagina of a woman for years, I still remembered what it felt like, and this just wasn't right. Not for me and not for her.

On my drive home from her house that first weekend, it hammered at me: *Could I have erectile dysfunction?* The precise words in my mind were less clinical, and certainly not as civil, but that was the bottom line. I think for the first time in my life I actually trembled with fear.

With erectile dysfunction, I faced the devastating prospect of never being able to give that special kind of pleasure that only an erect penis can deliver to a woman, and I would be deprived of the reciprocal joy as well.

With the feel of a woman in my arms with all those wonderful woman-parts to touch and taste, I could feel the feeling, the urge was powerful, but a solid erection evaded me. And each subsequent attempt just brought more angst and disappointment.

Over a period of months, we tried occasionally, but never with great success. She kept saying, "It's okay," and perhaps it was for her. She was older than I, past sixty, and maybe my companionship was more important to her than sex. But for me, I had gone a long time without. I wanted sex—great sex—and great sex is like a great dinner: It doesn't matter how fine the meal, or how elegant the restaurant, the next day you get hungry again.

I was starving, and I needed not just to perform, but to do so reliably and with mutual satisfaction.

Had it gone well, our affair might have lasted much longer. But it didn't. I got depressed and I got angry. Very angry in fact. Angry enough that my personality shifted and the relationship with my old lover deteriorated. Now I couldn't even keep female companionship which I also craved. I was a mess, but I've never been a quitter.

My Credentials

After getting my undergraduate degree in biology, I continued my studies and earned a Master's Degree in biochemistry and physiology. Studies in anatomy, immunology, and cell function all provided me with the disciplines required to understand the scientific basis of erectile dysfunction. I also have a foundation in statistics, specifically, the analysis of biological experimentation. That is, I can read a research paper and separate valid analyses from bullshit.

My second credential: I had ED.

I did research. The magnitude of the issue and the number of men who were suffering from erectile dysfunction was estimated in 2010 at 30,000,000–50,000,000 in the United States alone. This, of course, gave me no solace whatsoever. I didn't need a support group, and my misery didn't want company.

I was *single* again, and I wanted my old life back. I understood that as I approached sixty, even at full potency, the *me* of my thirties was ancient history. Still, I wanted to be capable of **sexual spontaneity** and to be fully confident when my opportunity to be a lover again came around.

I knew I wanted to do something about my ED, but I didn't know where to start. For reasons I will discuss later, I didn't want to rely on pills.

My "AHA!" Moment

Every night I was accosted by *those* commercials on TV. First there's the group of guys playing guitars and singing joyously about their flaccid dicks, and then you get to share the inane thoughts of some guy talking to his reflection in a store window about his limpy. A couple is painting a room that magically turns into a sex-garden. Every message is the same: the only solution is the quick-fix: pop a pill.

Then, there are the bathtubs. Will someone please explain the fucking bathtubs!

Each of these audiovisual abominations multiplied my indignation. Every program break assaulted me with some guy looking out from the screen all but directing his comments to me by name, mocking me.

A black man in his 50s confesses to the camera that he never realized that his diabetes could contribute to his erectile dysfunction. Another, a white guy about the same age, asks with sincerity, *Could my high blood pressure give me ED?*

I'm pathologically heterosexual, but I can still identify a guy who's got sex appeal to women. The commercials always feature great looking men. *If I looked like those guys*, I thought, *I'd get laid every night of the week.*

And then I realized, ***these guys are actors.*** They don't have diabetes or high blood pressure, and they're not likely candidates to ever get these diseases in real life. They are fit and trim with low body fat and ample musculature. They are youthful. While they have the bearing of men in their 50s, they exude an air of energy and vitality in contrast to most men with diabetes, high blood pressure, and erectile dysfunction who are out of shape, overweight, have poor skin tone, and generally look like shit.

Now, just as a disclaimer, doctors will rightly tell you that anyone can get diabetes or high blood pressure, fit or not, so get routine medical exams. But let's get real: out of a hundred men with these diseases, how many look like those guys on television, and how many look like that guy in your mirror? How flat is your stomach? Do you still have an ass? Might you be sporting a pouch like a turkey under your chin?

I asked myself the question: ***Does just being out-of-shape cause ED?***

Chapter 3: Initial Findings

In my research, I relied upon journal articles that had both scientific and statistical integrity. A growing number of younger men are experiencing erectile dysfunction. Obesity in that age range—as in all ages—is also increasing. But being a fat-ass doesn't automatically cause impotence. Regardless of how fat or fit they might be, percentage-wise, fewer guys under fifty experience ED than those over fifty. Then again, few young people who are heavy smokers get lung cancer and other pulmonary diseases compared to older folks.

And some people who smoke never get cancer. For all we know, they may not experience ED either.

Is it all genetic? Certainly that must be a factor. It is well established that those with a strong family history of cancer tend to get cancer more frequently, but usually of the same type—colon cancer leads to later generations with colon cancer, etc.—while families with a sporadic history as victims of disease, continue to have isolated occurrences in later generations. Up until *this* generation, of course. More about that later.

There just has to be something else operating.

From my research, I categorized sufferers of erectile dysfunction into four groups:

• Group 1: Men with a physical injury to the erection-producing apparatus, including, but not limited to, permanent nerve damage with or without prostate removal.

• Group 2: Men with a diagnosed biochemical source to their dysfunction, including, but not limited to, hormone issues.

These first two groups are states of dysfunction/disease for which medical alternatives are the best solution, if restoration of function is at all possible.

Then there are:

- Group 3: Those men whose ED is caused *primarily* by psychological factors.

- Group 4: Those guys who just have ED. Period. Their dicks don't work, or don't work well enough.

Group 4 is the largest and these are the men that I'll be primarily addressing in the remainder of this book. I'll also deal with Group 3 because as soon as any ED is suspected, a guy's psyche kicks into overdrive and makes things worse.

In the last several decades, much of the biochemistry of ED has been worked out by medical researchers, and this understanding has allowed the development of the medications now being prescribed at a cost to the healthcare system (public and private) of billions of dollars.

Science understands what's missing from the body that inhibits erections, and they've developed drugs to fill in the gaps. However, there is little discussion about where those missing pieces of the erectile puzzle have gone, and there's little or no attempt by the medical community to correct the problem. There's just no money in that.

What is it about the passage of years that causes half of all men over the age of sixty to have problems getting it up and keeping it up? Sure, the onset of other diseases may impact erectile function, but why do over a third of men in their fifties and sixties, who are otherwise disease-free, have ED?

I'm going to take you on a journey and lay out the product of my research in as direct a fashion as possible. So that you don't have to take notes, I tend to repeat some points as I go along when that information must be reapplied to a new topic.

Read it all. It will change the way you view your day to day treatment of your body.

Chapter 4: Dead Men Don't Get Laid

Erectile dysfunction can be a symptom of far more dangerous and life threatening diseases than just penile apathy. To eliminate the possibility that I was ill, I invested in a top-to-bottom medical examination. Along with the more general regimen of a physical, I had complete blood work performed, pulmonary testing, and an echocardiogram. As a man approaching sixty, I signed up for the beloved colonoscopy.

I spent about $2,000 out of pocket. I did not have insurance at the time and even if I did, other than my inability to sustain an erection, I had no physical complaints.

It was well worth the cost, if for no other reason than it confirmed what I had hoped; I was in pretty good physical condition, *by normal medical standards.* All I had to do was lose a few pounds—the doctor was being kind—and I would live forever.

My blood pressure was at the low end of the normal range. My cholesterol was on the high side of normal, but nowhere near dangerous levels; that was the only result about which my doctor cautioned me, and I immediately made some dietary adjustments to accommodate that finding.

My heart, lungs and blood work were all good. The internist who performed my colonoscopy told me that I was clean-as-a-whistle. I looked that up; it's not a medical term.

There was no reason for me to have erectile dysfunction, *by normal medical standards*. So, I was in Group 4, I had ED with no diagnosis, and I needed to find out why. My doctor couldn't tell me, because, *by normal medical standards,* health is just the absence of disease, and *that's just wrong*.

One cannot declare oneself *healthy* just because medical tests don't find anything overtly troublesome.

If you cannot walk a flight of stairs without becoming winded, or you have localized or generalized body pain for which a doctor cannot find a cause, then you're not healthy. You're just not necessarily *sick*.

"Hey, you're getting older," is not a diagnosis. It's a cop-out of the worst kind as it doesn't steer people in the direction of health. It gives them an alibi. Doctors should be ashamed of themselves when they advise their patients that they're just "old" regardless of how eloquently or humorously they may choose their words.

ED is not a disease of old age. It's a dysfunction with a reversible cause.

See Your Doctor Anyway

The average guy doesn't need medical permission to have sex, but if you have any ongoing issues, or if you suspect you may, or if you find yourself out-of-breath after simple exertion, or experience pains during or after exertion, then come on. Get real. Get a check-up.

Certainly, if you are having—or attempting to have—sex, and you begin to experience chest pains or the inability to breathe, call for help. Live to screw another day!

Throughout this book, I repeatedly emphasize that sex is an act of physical exertion that involves your heart, lungs, back and spine, along with the rest of your body, and that if you have, or suspect you might have, any condition that could be made worse by physical activity, speak to your doctor before engaging in sex.

Think about it. Even if you're lying flat, passively getting a hummer, by the time you climax, you're breathing is heavy, your heart is pounding, and you're in a mild sweat. And you haven't done anything except come! Sex is stressful even when you're not doing the work.

If you haven't had a complete checkup since you discovered you had erectile dysfunction, then get one. You must eliminate the possibility that a more serious issue is lurking in the wings.

PART II — Identifying the Problem & Seeking Solutions

Chapter 5: Why ED Drugs Are Not the Answer

In the early days of Viagra®, and with the release of each new ED medication, comedians and social commentators have gone over the top decrying the fact that doctors can't cure cancer, and engineers can't harness nature to produce clean, inexpensive energy, but the scientific community can, and does, devote its efforts and resources to rejuvenating dick.

We understand that ED does not just impair the lustful; it impacts couples who are deeply devoted and fully committed to each other, married couples and those in other life-long relationships. And ED affects women as much as men. No store-bought toy can take the place of a warm, hard, made-by-God penis that fits just right and is attached to her favorite handle—her man.

So, What's the Solution, If Not Drugs?

You know the names: Viagra® and Cialis® are the big guns and the most advertised products in the arena of erectile dysfunction, but there are others. Each has side effects—some severe—and each is contraindicated when you are taking certain other prescription medications that are frequently taken—not so coincidentally—by people who are getting on in years.

There is no certainty that ED drugs will work for one hundred percent of the men who take them, and no guarantee that they will work one hundred percent of the time on any individual man who has used them successfully. And like so many other drugs in conventional medicine, it just covers up the symptoms and doesn't address the underlying cause.

Drugs are a Band-Aid. They're something you might use as you work your wanger back to the land of the living. I did for a time, as a temporary fix, but you don't want to rely upon medications for the rest of your life.

Here are a couple of examples of why:

• Would you want an entire vacation ruined because you left one fucking little bottle of fucking pills back on the fucking bathroom counter? Fuck.

• A buddy sends a limo to pick you up so that you can attend a big party. You get in and realize that there's total privacy... just like in the movies! It's a 30 minute ride. Even if you had one with you, there's no time for a freaking pill to work.

Okay, this second scenario is far-fetched, but replace it with any opportunity that may arise—when you can't. Remember that time your woman raised her eyebrows, gave you that one special smile and said, "Wanna?" Do you want to say, "Sure. Let me take my pill and we'll wait half an hour and..."

Yeah, yeah, Cialis is advertising an "all the time" dose. In the next section, we'll discuss the downside of that, a $200+ monthly cost, plus Cialis' own warning: "Do not drink excessively when taking Cialis." What a buzz-kill.

There is No Such Thing as a "Side Effect"

There are *effects*. Just because the effect is not desired, or desirable, doesn't mean it's not an effect. When big pharmaceutical houses try to spin the possibly disastrous consequences of taking their drugs as side effects, they're asking you to "ignore the man behind the curtain."

The biochemistry of the human body is amazingly complex and efficient. Evolution continually borrowed working compounds from one part of the body and MacGyvered them for entirely different purposes in other places. Think about the cotter-pin. It held the wheel of a model-T on its axle, and now it's used to hold parts together on the military's most advanced stealth bombers.

Your body has done the same thing. Viagra and Cialis promote a biochemistry that gets you erect, but at the cost of other biochemical reactions all over your body. Many people get headaches with Cialis. Don't stand up too fast with either of these or you'll get lightheaded... if you don't pass out. And drink too much alcohol—is there such a thing?—and you could fall down without ever getting that erection.

As already stated, ED is often associated with *getting older.* So is high blood pressure, high cholesterol, and heart problems, and some of the drugs you will be forced to take to control these other life-threatening diseases won't permit you to take erectile dysfunction mediations. So what do you do? That's what the rest of this book is about.

The unintentional consequences of drugs—so called side-effects—aren't always apparent. Whatever Cialis does that can cause a headache in some men, it might be doing just a little in you. Not enough to give you a headache, but messing you up anyway. Even though you don't *feel* your oil running dry, that doesn't mean that at some point you're not going to throw a piston through your engine block. Get the idea?

If there's a way to resolve your erectile dysfunction, high blood pressure, diabetes, asthma, or other allergies without drugs, you've just gotta try, always, of course, keeping your physician in the loop.

Chapter 6: How Happy Harry Happens

Second only to the vagina, there can be no more perfect biological element on the planet than the human penis. Penile plumbing is a wonder of hydraulics. That it gets as hard and resistant to bending as it does—who of us didn't test that as a kid—is amazing, and it's all about fluid pressure. When you'd delve into the complex biochemistry, neurology, and physiology of an erection, you're likely astonished that it ever works at all!

Pressure in the penis is regulated by both the inflow and outflow of blood. There are two separate channels, one for blood in and one for blood out.

Arteries and their smaller brethren, arterioles, carry blood from the heart via a branching tree of vessels to organs throughout the body, including the penis. Venules and veins carry the blood back toward the heart.

Interestingly, a resting penis is regulated by an active function. Smooth muscles in the walls of the arterioles leading into the penis are contracted, constricting blood flow. They allow only enough blood into Harry to keep him alive and breathing, but not quite awake.

When chilled, as when one is swimming in cold water, these small vessels contract even further, and the reduction of normal blood flow that this constriction causes, results in the now infamous, but very real condition of "shrinkage."

For a penis to become erect there must be a stimulus—physical or mental—that sets off a series of signals from the brain down to the fun factory. Neurotransmitters tell the smooth muscle of the arteries to relax and blood begins to flow filling the spongy material of the shaft of the penis, the corpus spongiosum—or *spongecake* as my spell checker insists—and the corpus cavernosa. You gotta love how they named these things.

Blood is pumped in at an increasingly higher pressure. At the same time, the smooth muscles in the walls of the veins that carry blood out of the penis are constricted. This traps the blood inside. Pressure builds and Harry rises to the occasion.

The guy has to stay that way for some period of time while you satisfy your lady and yourself. Sometime after ejaculation—depending on your age and state of inebriation—the process reverses; the veins open allowing blood out, while the arteries constrict preventing much blood from entering. Harry slumbers off.

Nitric Oxide—Part I

Hormones play a major role in the control of male sexual function just as they do in women. Behind all the mechanics, there is a biochemistry to creating an erection, sustaining an erection, achieving ejaculation, and the desire for a drink afterwards.

However, a discussion of this biochemistry is far beyond the scope of this presentation; it's unnecessary to simplify the elaborately complex process to fit into the context of this discussion. But introducing you to a simple little control molecule is key.

Nitric oxide (chemical formula: NO—one Nitrogen atom attached to one Oxygen atom) does much of the heavy lifting when it comes to snapping Harry to attention. Viagra® does its magic primarily by increasing the amount of NO in your pecker. Cialis® does too, though by a mechanism different from Viagra.

Special Note: Nitric Oxide, NO, which is essential for erections, is not the same a Nitrous Oxide, NO_2 (one Nitrogen atom and TWO Oxygen atoms), which is used most commonly by dentists as a pain killer—laughing gas.

Nitric Oxide is a vasodilator; it opens blood vessels allowing increased flow. You can see how this is essential to opening that inflow artery to pump up the volume. It is produced throughout the body. When you exercise, blood vessels need to dilate—become larger in diameter—to deliver more blood to muscles. The cells at the interior walls of blood vessels produce the nitric oxide they need. Healthy vessels produce a lot in a constant stream which keeps arteries and veins working efficiently.

Have you ever become flushed with embarrassment or rage? Same thing. The quantity of nitric oxide increases in the vessels of your face, and you go red.

As you age, the lining of your blood vessels deteriorate from the cumulative abuse of years of exposure to inflammatory chemicals, poor nutrition, and crap food. Your vessels' ability to produce nitric oxide declines. Hence—in part—the correlation between age and ED. But it's reversible.

Disease conditions such as high blood pressure beat the hell out of your blood vessels with a concomitant reduction in their ability to produce nitric oxide. We'll speak more about this in our discussion of inflammation.

It must be noted that overarching all this is an extensive neural network. Nerves carry stimulation from your genitals to your brain, and transmit the brain's commands back to Harry's control mechanisms.

The Three EDs

There are three kinds of erectile dysfunction. The unusual names I use to describe these three conditions should make you aware that these have not yet been fully accepted by the larger sphere of the scientific or medical community:

• First, the type of ED that keeps one from getting an erection at all—the *Limpy*. If there's some stiffness, it's not enough to penetrate a vagina, even if she's hungry.

• Second, there's the *Transitory Stiffy*. Things start out well, but begin to wane even while you're inside and feeling good. It goes away before either of you are satisfied. It may or may not come back during that session.

• Finally, there's Bonehead, your guy seems to forget why he's there. You're stiff enough—perhaps just barely so—but not rock-hard. Still, you can keep things going. You just can't cross the finish line. You can't ejac, Jack. Candidly, this isn't actually ED, it's a condition called anorgasmy/anejaculation, but it may have some neurological relation to ED, so I'm going to include it in our discussion.

The reasons for the onset of each of these EDs are varied and often a product of more than one cause.

If Bonehead isn't caused psychologically, it might be attributed to a reduction in the sensation during sex. For example, the loss of direct contact when one uses a condom makes it more difficult for even some younger men to achieve climax. Imagine a reduction in sensation that makes you feel as if you're wearing a condom all the time.

There can be other factors. Contemporary media has made a cliché of "size matters." The clear implication is that a man with a large penis is more desirable and satisfying to a woman than a man with a normal or small organ inasmuch as a mega-wanger gives her a greater *sensation of presence* during sex and concomitant pleasure. The key factor, guys, is width, not length, but since one usually occurs with the other, well...

However, "size matters" ignores the corresponding female affliction: the Bell-Jar Vagina.

After birthing a few kids and through the normal action of hormone rearrangement and age, the muscles of vaginae (yep, that's the plural) tend to weaken. There's also a reduction in the engorgement of female erectile tissue, something I won't discuss here much beyond the observation that this tissue contributes to "tightness," in the absence of which, in simple terms, the cavity gets larger.

A regularly hung guy just can't reasonably fill the void. Sure, there's contact, but not the kind she offered in her youth. If you're using an artificial lubricant or if your woman naturally lubricates too well, then there just isn't sufficient friction and therefore not enough sensation to bring you off.

This same female condition can also contribute to a Transitory Stiffy. Loss of erection can occur during sex just because you're not getting enough "rub." If you're using a condom, you might as well phone it in.

Match a guy with some reduced sensitivity issues and a bell-jar woman and there had better be a liberal use of alternate methods to achieve and sustain arousal or little is going to happen.

The Transitory Stiffy (TS) proves that—at the very least—the basic plumbing works. Loss of erection can occur if the exit valve, the muscles in the veins that retain blood in your penis, are not being controlled properly or are too weak and tire quickly. This can, in some instances, be a "true" dysfunction; the valve mechanism may be damaged or, in rare cases, malformed congenitally. Even small deviations from optimal formation of the valve can be exaggerated by the progression of years. At some point it just doesn't work anymore—the muscles within the veins fail after a short period of contraction. There may be a surgical fix for this, but it is best if, failing the suggestions in this book, you discuss that with your urologist.

Or the wiring—the nerves that control the erectile function—may not be performing. We'll speak about this in much greater detail later on.

Combine some blood pressure control issues with some loss of sensitivity and TS can easily manifest.

The Limpy. Once you've eliminated any clinical issues by subjecting yourself to a thorough examination by a urologist...

Joke Time: A guy goes to his urologist. He's led to an examining room where, a few minutes later, a gorgeous, blue-eyed blond walks in. She's sporting a stethoscope around her neck that rests enviably on her ample bosom. Noticing the guy's confusion, she explains, "I'm your urologist. I'm working with Dr. Smith and I am Board Certified. I've been practicing for several years and I assure you I've seen it all. Please don't be embarrassed to discuss your issue with me. What is your problem?" "Well, Doc," the man says, "my dick tastes funny."

So, you've got a Limpy. You go to your urologist and she can't find anything physiologically wrong. You have to consider one of a few alternatives. Your doctor will undoubtedly suggest counseling— she may want you to consider that your ED may be psychological, and that may be true. But there are other reasons you can't get it up.

You're Group 4. We'll review these conditions as we go along: severe manifestation of poor lymph drainage, neural inflammations and nutritional deficits.

Chapter 7: Gut Feelings

So far, I've discussed why the topic of erectile dysfunction is important to me, and what motivated me to seek the answer to my dilemma. I've described my reasoning for not wanting to settle for the pill-popping quick-fix as a way of life. We've also reviewed the control mechanisms that prime Harry for the deed.

Now, I'm going to share with you what I discovered as I dug into the medical and anecdotal research.

Rowing Down the Alimentary Canal

Your alimentary canal is a tube running from your mouth to your butt. Digestion begins in the mouth, but the major digestive area includes the stomach, the small intestine and the large intestine (bowel). This is also called the gastrointestinal (GI) tract.

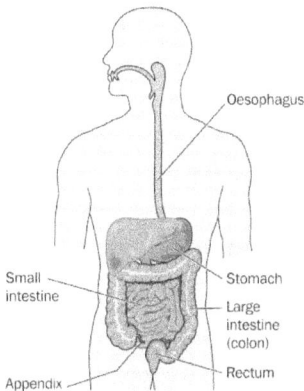

There is a school of thought, predominantly among alternative medical practitioners, that most disease starts in the GI tract. Because the primary purpose of these organs is digestion, digestive disorders are the cause of most bodily problems, and erectile dysfunction is no exception.

Diet: a Definition

Before going any further, I'd like to define the word "diet." This word has taken on the connotation of what we restrict from our food mix to accomplish a goal such as weight loss, a better state of health, or generally just to make ourselves miserable.

Dictionary.com defines diet as *"food and drink considered in terms of its qualities, composition, and its effects on health..."* In fact we are all on a diet all the time. Sometimes it's a healthy diet and all too often it's putting us on a path to make us ill and dysfunctional. It's in this sense that I'm going to use the word.

Are you eating well? Your body tells you every day, and it does so by what it passes out.

The Answer My Friend is Blowin' in the Wind

Let's first address flatulence—farts, that is. We are all familiar with the scene in the college movie. *Animal House* had such a scene, but it surely was not unique to that flick. Five guys are riding in a car—road trip. The guy in the middle of the back seat, usually a really fat guy, lets loose with a resonant explosion. The others start waving their hands and hanging out the windows and, of course, all the boys in the audience who are under the age of eleven—perhaps mentally so—laugh hysterically.

The question is, are all farts that noxious? The answer, obviously, is no. Even those people who often leave a bathroom so pungent that the wallpaper peels, aren't that odoriferous all the time; they have good days and bad days. But why are some people often passing farts that violate the Geneva Convention's ban on chemical weapons?

Farts are expelled gas. Some of it is swallowed air that gets pushed along through the alimentary canal all the way to the end. Most of it is a byproduct of the biochemistry of the digestive process, the result of what bacteria in our intestines do to the food we eat. Those bacteria are an important part of converting food into a form that our bodies can absorb for nutrition; we need the bacteria, and we need much of what they produce.

Sometimes food is digested well and that will result in sweet farts that are barely noticeable. Too often, food is digested poorly allowing putrefaction: rotting. The food in your gut rots like road-kill. The result is the kind of smell that is best described by the diatribe, "What crawled up your ass and died?" It's no joke, except that it climbed down through your mouth and you put it there.

What goes in must come out. The canal from mouth to butt is a continuous tube and many things happen to our food along the way. It's mixed with enzymes in the mouth, acids in the stomach, and more digestive juices as it moves through the small intestine.

We need a balance of protein, fat, starch, carbohydrates, fiber, vitamins, minerals, and other nutrients. Humans are omnivores; we can eat everything, and we should. One source of the fart problem is an imbalance in the proportions of these "food groups" in our diet.

The fiber in vegetable matter is essential to move other food through the GI tract at a reasonable rate. Meat and potato guys— those that get very little green vegetable matter—tend to have stronger smelling farts. In the absence of fiber, the movement of food slows so that there's time for it to rot in your gut, and the raunchiest smells possible begin to emanate from your ass.

Regardless of the social aspects of flatulence, what comes out of your body is an indication of what's happening inside.

Unless you want to die while still too young to have enjoyed all the sex there is to be had, you must address digestive issues early on. Colon cancer is rising to epidemic proportions in the West largely due to the reduction of fiber in the American diet, and yet, we keep making fart jokes.

Think I Don't Know Shit? Well, I Do

All kidding aside, those terribly bad smells are an indication that something is wrong in your digestion. And that takes us to the next topic: Poop.

Author's Note: I use the word "poop" because "shit" is what you say when you get a flat on your way to a hot date, and "crap" is what you look like when you show up late, sweaty and greasy from changing the tire.

You eat two or three times a day. You should have at least one decent dump a day. Maybe two. And every day. Dropping a few rabbit pellets for a couple of days followed by one big catch-up load is not healthy.

Keeping the contents of your bowels moving will prolong the quality of your life and perhaps life itself. As I've already said, colon cancer is getting more common. Statistically, deaths from colon cancer may not be increasing as much as one might expect; this is due to advances in detection and surgical removal of the effected organ, but you just don't want to tempt the fates by allowing bad eating habits to get those parasitic cells growing in your body.

Colon surgery isn't fun. The recovery isn't fun. And you won't get laid for months while you're healing. This kind of surgery saves your life, but it also ages you! Aging reduces your useful sex life. Get the point?

So, eat every day; poop every day. If you have eaten a big meal, or meals, then expect to poop more. If you pig out at the all-you-can-eat buffet on Saturday, and you don't have a commensurate dump on Sunday, then the train has stopped in the station too long; you've gotta eat some veggies.

Fiber is the key to creating a steady flow through your bowels. It is an indigestible component of plants. Animals don't produce it. You must eat plant matter to get it. Fiber is essential to your bowel health. There are two types: soluble and insoluble. The flesh of fruit is the soluble kind; it forms a gel when mixed with water. The firmer type, like the stalks of celery and broccoli, is insoluble. You need both.

Soluble fiber mops up a lot of excess stuff in your digestive tract. It will adhere to harmful components of our diets. Like throwing sand on an oil-spot on your garage floor, soluble fiber will cling onto some harmful substances, and carry them out the back door. Insoluble fiber creates bulk and just keeps things moving.

A Well-Formed Stool is Not a Wood Shop Project

Your dumps should be real dumps. You shouldn't be shooting hard little billiard balls off the porcelain. Nor should you feel like a soft-serve machine. Most of the time you should be passing what medical doctors call a "well-formed stool."

Made famous by Bill Murray's character Carl Spackler in *Caddy Shack*, a well-formed stool should look like a Babe Ruth bar with tapered ends.

Color is important, too. If your stools are black, I mean real black, you may have a serious digestive issue and you should see your physician immediately.

Poop should be brown, a product of the color of bile (yellow) acted on by digestive enzymes. If your stools are too yellow for a long period of time, again, see your doctor; there may be too much bile or a clinical issue that causes improper digestion upstream.

Along with the metabolic remains of last night's dinner, poop also contains a considerable volume of bacterial cells and dead cells from the walls of your digestive tract.

The question arises: while you are digesting a cow's meat, why aren't you digesting the meat that is you? Answer: your stomach and intestines are lined with mucous which protects your body from being processed along with the Porterhouse. This protection is not perfect and digestion takes a toll. Many cells are shed from the lining of your GI tract along the way. These add up. So, even when your schedule puts you in a situation where "I've hardly eaten anything for the past two days," if your digestion is working properly, you should still have bowel movements.

And Then There's Pee

Since the beginning of medical science, physicians have recognized that one's urine can tell much regarding the state of one's health. Before modern chemical testing, doctors would smell and taste their patients' urine. If it was sweet, there would be a presumption of diabetes. If it smelled musty, it could be a sign of liver or other metabolic disorders.

Note: if you think that's disgusting, it's just the *yuk* factor. In a healthy individual, urine is sterile, containing no bacteria, viruses, or health risk to another person.

Short lived changes in smell and color are to be expected. If you eat asparagus, excess asparagine, an amino acid present in significant quantities in the vegetable, will pass through you quickly and be eliminated within hours. You will smell the distinctive odor when you urinate and should not be alarmed.

Foul smelling urine—not just a strong smell—may be a sign of a urinary tract infection and should be addressed with your physician immediately.

Normally, your urine should be light yellow with little objectionable smell. Very dark urine is an indication that you are dehydrated; you should drink a glass or two or water immediately and increase your water intake until it lightens.

Drink only pure, clean water. Caffeine and certain other components of sport drinks and sodas are diuretics; they make you pee and dehydrate you even more. Alcohol also causes diuresis; remember the saying "You don't buy beer, you only rent it." You're not just getting rid of the beer, you're also dumping a lot of additional water from your system. Dehydration is the major cause of hangover nausea and headaches.

Taking vitamins or mixed nutritional supplements will also change your urine color and smell. The B vitamins are notorious for this. Excess B's will pass through you faster than the Mayor of Hiroshima could say, "What was that?"

After taking vitamins, if you haven't eaten, you could be seeing orange, pungent Vit B pee within an hour. Make sure you're reasonably hydrated; you don't want any crystals—stones—forming in your kidneys or bladder.

Unless you drink water throughout the night, your first pee upon waking should be the strongest—darkest and most odoriferous—of your day.

Burps & Belches

If you're digesting poorly, sometimes the smell that accompanies a belch can be, for all practical purposes, indistinguishable from what comes out of your ass, and can fill a confined space with the same noxious effect. Healthier digestion reduces the burp to just what you've eaten recently.

Eat slower, swallow less air, and drink less, especially reduce carbonated drinks with your meals.

The Little Greek Whore

Joke Time: Medieval age—an adviser leans toward the Queen while the King is addressing the court, "M'lady, the Kings's mouth smells of halitosis." The Queen sighs and asks, "Was that little Greek whore here again?"

Poor digestion can cause bad breath. Bad breath is a direct cause of loneliness. All the mouthwash and breath mints you might use cannot remove the odor of those smells that emanate from your lungs and stomach even when you have not belched.

Poor digestion can result in this singularly most socially unacceptable condition. Further, poor digestion from bad food combination can also modify your overall biochemistry to promote dental issues including, but not limited to, gum disease and, consequently, even worse breath.

Eat more green and colored, non-starchy vegetables, drink pure clean water, avoid mixing meat and dairy, and balance your meals with members of all the food groups.

The most direct cause of halitosis is poor dental hygiene and gum disease. Periodontal inflammation and infection can also result in poor overall health. Juices from chewed vegetables, especially greens rich in chlorophyll, wash gums and kill germs, improving gum and tooth health, and one's breath.

And a note on smoking: the act of simply breathing can bring up a smell from your lungs as repulsive as an ashtray full of cigarette butts. Women and men both tend to breathe in just before they kiss. First, a long kiss might require a little extra oxygen. Second, evolutionarily, each is "breathing the other in," detecting pheromones. These are sex hormones that identify the other as chemically "attractive" or not. If the strong smell of tobacco from your lungs is lingering on your breath, she will quickly shut down... even if she also smokes.

Your Sweat Stinks, Too!

Your skin is an organ of excretion. Bad nutrition will have an impact on what comes out of your sweat glands as it does with all the other holes in your body.

It's not just about arm pits. Almost every inch of you, especially your groin, excretes perspiration that is filled with the byproducts of your metabolism. Bacteria that naturally inhabit the warm, wet folds of your body—pits, groin, butt—begin to act on the chemicals discharged by your sweat glands immediately upon its arrival at the surface of your skin. This bacterial action causes the usual body odor associated with being sweaty.

For several hours after a great, refreshing shower, you should be odor free. It takes some time for bacteria to gear up and process your sweat and oily secretions of your skin. However, if your freshly washed body still had body-odor, it's from the waste products of your bodily processes.

Sweat glands discharge the chemical remains of bad nutrition. Without being sweaty, you will give off a body odor of the most alienating kind.

Women have an exceptionally keen olfactory sense. That is, besides smelling good, they smell well. They can detect when you're covering up a smelly body with even the most evocative store-bought body scent.

Man-rule: It is impossible to own body-wash and testicles at the same time. Men use soap.

So, you make incredible, acrobatic, sweaty love and collapse into her arms in exhaustion during the night. Do you want her to cringe in disgust when she wakes up in the morning breathing in the smell of a glue-factory? It could put a kibosh on your sunrise wake-up call... and we do love our sunrise wake-up calls. This is yet another reason to get your nutrition and digestion in balance.

Thanks for staying with me as I surveyed what comes out of your body. Some of you may have found it amusing. I hope you all found it informative. Everything here applies equally to women, so let her know about this, too.

Chapter 8: Eat, Drink, and Be Harry

Anthelme Brillat-Savarin was a French lawyer and politician. In December, 1825, he published his tome *The Physiology of Taste*. In it he included the aphorism "Tell me what kind of food you eat, and I will tell you what kind of man you are." Several decades later, German philosopher and anthropologist Ludwig Andreas Feuerbach penned, "Man is what he eats." This phrase has been handed down to us more generalized as "You are what you eat."

No rational person would argue that a diet high in fat and cholesterol, fried foods, sweets and pastries is healthy. As the years progress, this kind of diet will lead to obesity and a serious degradation of one's health. This is especially true for those people who also slow down and begin to spend fewer and fewer hours each week in physical activity. These guys are destined to become card-carrying couch potatoes in their sixties… fifties… forties?

Our predilection for insanely loud music in our youth has ramifications for our hearing later in life. Similarly, poor diet does some invisible and asymptomatic damage to our blood vessels and nerves when we are young. As we pass fifty and head for sixty, this predisposes us to health issues including, but not limited to, erectile dysfunction.

Not a damn thing we can do about it now that we're here. What is, is. The good news is that this predisposition is not a jail sentence. With improved respect for our bodies, we can still rescue our hearts, lungs, colons, and dicks from incarceration and put them on parole. Perhaps we can get them an outright pardon.

Depending on your current mix of healthy versus crap food, you will have to adjust proportions. In extreme cases, you may have to reduce the intake of some favorites to the point they are considered rare treats.

This chapter focuses on a number of topics that are important to your health, including erectile function, but not tied point-by-point to getting Harry back online. Read it. It will answer many questions including some you may not have thought of. It illustrates how, with each eating and drinking decision you make, you can reduce the dick-softening chemicals from your daily consumption. Remember: Erectile Dysfunction is the *cumulative effect* of all the offenders you eat, drink, and think (the last point to be considered later).

We'll discuss:

- Food quality
- Organic food
- A dispensation for eating fat
- An admonition to avoid Fluoride in water and elsewhere
- A few other topics

Food Quality

You trash your body with fried, greasy, crap food. That abuse filters down to your pecker. Flip side: embarking on a program to improve your overall health makes its way to Harry & Co. as well.

Earlier, I used the B-word—broccoli—and implied that this vegetable along with others like it will confer an overall health benefit. If you still have kids living under your roof, it could help them, too; if Dad starts eating healthier, the kids just might join you.

Do it for the kids, man, do it for the kids!

What's really a shame is that when you decide to exert all the effort and willpower to finally clean up your act, eat healthier, attacking the root cause of your ED and other health issues, you get caught in the nightmare of corporate greed.

Huh? What?

The quality of the food in the United States has drastically deteriorated in the past fifty years. The trend downward has accelerated in the last decade. I'm not speaking of the taste. I'm referring to the intrinsic nutritional content of the foodstuffs provided by commercial sources. What you see on your supermarket shelves and in produce department bins is not necessarily what you think you're getting.

We'll stay with broccoli; it's a great example of what you may run into with every trip to the supermarket. But these cautions apply to most foods you buy, especially packaged and prepared items.

Broccoli is naturally high in calcium. Kids need calcium to grow, and mature women need calcium to deter the onset of osteoporosis, so this vegetable is commonly referenced in the media.

Calcium figures in generalized good health, so men should have a regular dose of calcium via broccoli or other cruciferous vegetables throughout the week. Calcium is an element—number 20 on the Periodic Chart—that is found in the soil. Calcium is not produced by the broccoli plant. It has to be absorbed through its roots from the soil. Calcium has to be in the soil for it to be absorbed by the roots of the broccoli plant. Got that?

After a few seasons of growing broccoli in a field, it absorbs all the calcium from the soil; the soil becomes depleted. The soil runs out. There is no more. The soil is *sans* calcium.

Large agribusinesses, the producers of most of the fresh and frozen vegetables in this country, grow, harvest, package, and distribute millions of tons of fresh looking and delectable fruits and vegetables each year. It is expensive to put calcium in the soil to be absorbed so that the broccoli that you're forcing down your throat actually has calcium in it. It costs the agribusinesses millions to ensure that calcium, along with other nutrients and trace minerals essential to your health, are in the soil.

Often agribusinesses don't go that extra mile to ensure that the plants they're growing have a complete complement of nutritional ingredients, calcium being just one of many. Even if they do, they use synthetic fertilizers as opposed to natural ones which introduce other issues.

You wind up with beautiful looking broccoli that just doesn't have an adequate quantity of calcium for you to go through all the effort of convincing yourself it tastes good. You're being ripped off.

More: good agricultural husbandry calls for leaving fields fallow—not used—for periods of time and rotating crops. This understanding goes so far back that it's mentioned in the Bible. But it's costly and rarely practiced as thoroughly as it should by the ever-so-cost-conscious businesses that run our major food delivery systems *for* this country. Please take note that I deliberately say "...FOR this country," and not "IN" this country because so much of what we put in our mouths and our bodies comes from somewhere outside the United States and Canada.

As agribusiness looks for lower and lower costs to increase their profits, they don't exercise the degree of oversight we consumers would expect—demand?—regarding how our food is handled when grown off-shore. Wiki "night soil."

There is a benefit to eating broccoli even if it has been grown in soil that is low in calcium. First, there's always some small amount of calcium or the plant just wouldn't grow; it needs it, too. Second, the makeup of the plant is roughage and contributes to your fiber requirement for bowel health. Third, if you're filling up on broccoli you're not eating crap food.

You're going to all the trouble of buying, preparing, and eating broccoli. Why not get the most bang for the buck at the dinner table which will also give you the most bang when you're the buck in the bedroom?

Building on this understanding, there is something you can do immediately—TODAY—to bring Harry back to life:

Eat healthier and cleaner versions of the food you're already eating.

What the Hell is Organic Food Anyway?

Let's clear our plate of the pesticide issue. Agribusinesses can't afford to have crops destroyed—and suffer financial losses—due to insect infestation. They spray insecticides on their produce in the fields. These poisons are absorbed into the plants and wind up on your dinner plate. Don't believe anyone that tells you that pesticides are safe for humans and only kill bugs. That's a lie. *People who apply pesticides to crops wear hazmat suits.*

Most people have the misconception that food grown organically is merely produced without pesticides. This is only part of a much larger story.

"Organically-grown fruits and vegetables obtain their nutrients from healthy soils, rather than synthetic fertilizers. They are lower in water content, thus preserving a higher nutrient density, they are richer in iron, magnesium, vitamin C, and antioxidants, and they provide a more balanced combination of essential amino acids."

This excerpt is from IFOAM.org, the web site of the International Federation of Organic Agricultural Movements. The most comprehensive page on their web site that describes the advantages of organically grown foods can be found in **Links & References**.

From that same page regarding animal products:

"Organic livestock farmers work to optimize the animals' health and well-being, rather than maximizing their potential output, through rearing practices, such as a balanced diet and sufficient room for physical and mental needs.

"Organically-raised animals have better overall health, especially in the areas of reproduction and recovery from illness. Organically-raised animals have a reduced risk of carrying diseases, in fact, no record of BSE [Bovine spongiform encephalopathy—mad cow, or Denny Crane's disease] has been found in organically-raised animals.

Organically-raised animals have an ideal fat profile, that is, they have a lower ratio of saturated to unsaturated fat."
([ ] added by author)

Hormone-free and antibiotic-free meats, free-range chicken eggs, breads, butter, and cheese are all available as organic. Most of the snack foods you look forward to are available as organic, too. Understand that organic potato chips are still potato chips—fried starch. But at least if there's any nutrition to a potato chip at all, you'll get it in the organic version, and you won't be getting the poisons associated with tainted farm products.

This discussion is just a brief snippet regarding organics. Many people don't incorporate organic foods into their weekly shopping because of the cost. It is more costly to grow food under the precepts of organic agriculture, and those costs have to be passed on to you as the consumer.

However, the gap in prices has dropped as greater numbers of people buy these cleaner and healthier versions of the same foods they've enjoyed all along. Increased demand has led to increased production and diversity of offerings. Supermarket chains have sprung up to meet these demands. Organic food will likely remain a tad more expensive, but the margin will close further.

Chicken: an example of quality lost

At one time, chicken soup used to be called Jewish penicillin. In a traditional Jewish household, whenever someone got a cold, the flu, or was just under-the-weather, a pot of chicken soup would be cooked up and distributed, not just to the afflicted individual, but to everyone in the home. Non-Jewish neighbors benefited from it, too.

Funny thing is, it actually worked.

This is so well established in American culture that Jack Canfield and Mark Victor Hanson (funny, they don't look Jewish) sold over a hundred million books franchising the "Chicken Soup for the..." concept.

How does chicken soup reduce the severity and shorten the lifetime of a cold?

Back in the old country—Eastern Europe and Russia—chickens were easy to raise. They provided both eggs and meat to poor farmers in small towns. The chickens were allowed to roam free and they would eat bugs and critters along with seeds and other vegetation. Chickens, like us, are omnivores; they'll eat anything.

The proteins and other compounds that make up bugs are very healthy for chickens. Chicken metabolism converts these raw materials into other proteins and compounds that are very healthy for us. These healthy materials are stored and concentrated, to a large extent, *in the fat of the chicken.*

Back in those days, and up until the 1960s, chicken fat— *schmaltz,* in Yiddish—was used extensively in Jewish homes, basically the same as pork fat is so often incorporated into cooking by non-Jewish families.

The fat left in the soup conferred the health-given and cold-curing effects of chicken soup.

Two things have happened in the past four decades. First, agribusiness has all but eliminated the free-roaming chicken that eats bugs, in favor of the more profitable caged animals that are fed a diet of lesser nutritional value. No bugs, no penicillin.

Second, fat has been demonized. Even in Jewish households, often the layer of fat that floats to the surface of a pot of chicken soup as it cools is skimmed off and discarded; any remaining health benefit that the fat may contain goes down the garbage disposal.

Chickens raised under the organic umbrella, are free-range. They eat bugs. They grow some extra fat on their bodies. They're happy. *Within reasonable limits*, we should enjoy the taste, texture and health benefits of their fat.

Fat is Okay

Fat by itself is not unhealthy. The fat/cholesterol scare was manufactured through faulty science in the 1950s and has been debunked. Never buy low-fat anything because ironically, by taking out the fat, room is made for more harmful substances to take its place.

Still, *excess* fat is not healthy for two reasons:

- Fat does not automatically glom onto your waistline; fat doesn't directly convert to fat on your body. But fat has more than twice the calories of protein or carbohydrates. If you're trying to lose weight, *excess* fat in your diet will slow your weight-loss.
- Many harmful environmental chemicals are fat soluble; they concentrate in the fat of animals that have, for example, been fed pesticide-laden grain. Eating non-organic animal fat contributes to your toxic load.

Cut down on carbohydrates as they pose a greater direct health risk, not from their caloric content, but from what they do biochemically in the body. I won't discuss the topic here, but you can Google "Hyperinsulinism" or "Insulin resistance," or visit my blog, *http://NutritionalLeverage.com* to read more.

The takeaway: non-fat or low-fat foods are not healthier alternatives to their full-fat versions. In dairy products, they're less healthy.

Locally-Grown

A less expensive compromise to organic is *locally-grown* produce which is more likely to have higher vitamin and enzyme concentrations; the food has not traveled as far and is offered at the store much sooner after it has been harvested.

When I see that an organic cucumber costs $2.00, I amble over to the locally-grown section of the produce department and pick one up for $0.69 or less.

Enzymes are temperature and time labile. That means when exposed to changes in temperature or just over time, they degrade, even while still in the vegetables and fruits. It's basic to healthy eating to consume produce as soon after harvest as possible. If you already enjoy these foods, purchase locally grown to save money and ensure high enzyme and nutritional potency. The only thing better is growing them yourself.

Why does this matter? ***Nutritional potency helps your potency.***

Two generations ago, everyone ate organic food. Prior to DDT and other manufactured pesticides, most of the food grown in this country was produced without chemicals and only natural fertilizers were added to the fields. It was all grown locally. Importing food from other countries, even shipping from distant parts of this country, was costly; for some products it was totally impractical. There were a greater number of small, local farms and dairies from which individuals and markets could purchase food. The latter supplied this nutritious produce for sale to the public. Such was the age before multinational agribusiness which has all but eliminated the family-owned farm in the United States.

Even if these profit hungry monsters were entirely on-board with organic agriculture, the way they are organized prevents delivery of produce and animal products that retain all that nature has provided in live enzymes and other essential compounds.

A glimmer of hope: there are a growing number of local food cooperatives being formed in both urban and suburban areas that provide locally grown AND organic food to members. Google "organic food co-op [your city]" to find one. If there is none, form one.

Author's note: Saturday morning farmers' markets are a great place to meet women.

It is essential to align yourself with one of these groups. Next Halloween, if you wish to watch a movie that will truly scare the living shit out of you, watch *The Future of Food*.

I began eating salads as part of my quest to resurrect Harry, but I'm not a zealot. I purchase as much organically grown food as I can afford and is reasonably available. I will not starve myself in the absence of an organic version of food I enjoy. I still eat pizza and Chinese food in restaurants, the sources of the ingredients being entirely unknown to me.

However, **whatever the incrementally higher cost of organic food may be, it is not as expensive as the ED drugs or the co-pay on medical insurance.** While the drugs have negative side effects, eating cleaner, healthier organic food has important and powerful positive effects on vitality and longevity in the bedroom and out.

I try to eat a salad, even a small one, every day. Sometimes I miss a day here and there. When I do, I don't stress-out or beat myself up about it (much more about stress later). I believe a healthy lifestyle, good food choices, and a reasonable amount of exercise is as much an art as a science.

When I do eat salad, I try to use only organic leafy greens including some of those purple ones. Iceberg lettuce, even if organically grown, has very little nutrition and should be replaced with romaine lettuce or "baby herbs." You'll see them labeled that way on the store shelf. Spinach has an ANDI score [discussed next] of about 700, out of 1000, and should be included with your salad greens.

I add some organic carrots and some olives and cucumber. I usually slice a hardboiled egg—an omega-3 or free-range egg—and put that on top. Optionally, I add toasted croutons (rarely organic), and use a modicum of organic salad dressing

Recently, I started adding diced red, yellow, and occasionally orange bell peppers to my salad. Their sweetness makes it enjoyable without the salad dressing.

I never use anything with hydrogenated oils or trans-fats. I mean as close to NEVER as is humanly possible. When purchasing packaged foods, I read the label; if it has "partially hydrogenated oils"—the notorious *trans-fats*—I put it back on the shelf. We all get enough of these poisons on those occasions when we eat junk-food at the fast-food toxinary.

I'm convinced that the long-term use of these manufactured ingredients goes right to Harry. What constitutes long-term is the question: a year, a month, four or five days in a row? I don't know. Why take the chance? They're just not good for your dick or anything that's attached to it.

Surely, some of you may ask, "When I was in my twenties, I ate all the crap in the world and I could still screw like an 18V DeWalt. What's the big deal?"

The answer is simple. It's the cumulative effect of bad eating over the decades that cause Harry to punk-out as we pass fifty. It's the assault of these poisons on our bodies that overwhelm our aging digestive systems that make us ill. Just one symptom of this abuse is a hapless Harry.

ANDI Score?

You'll see ANDI scores or simply "Nutrient Density" numbers associated with produce at health food markets.

Average Nutrient Density Index: Promoted and described by Dr. Joel Fuhrman in his book *Eat for Health*, it's a way of comparing foods based on their nutrient density per calorie; this is the amount of actual health-promoting nutrients you get relative to the number of calories you consume.

Kale is indexed at 1000 and is the highest. It's the basis for the entire index—like batting 1000. Spinach is about 700 and is great for bowel health as well. Popeye wouldn't lie.

The higher the ANDI score the better, but it's just an index. If you don't like kale, as I don't, eat spinach or some other leafy green. Don't take ANDI too seriously. You know that salads are healthier than potatoes; you don't need a chart to figure that out.

It's Not Just the Food We Eat

Do you drink pure, clean water? In an age when multinational food companies—some of those same companies to which I've referred in the last section—fill potentially toxic plastic bottles with water from hoses behind their manufacturing plant and sell them for a dollar a piece—okay, that may be an exaggeration, or not—and nippled bottles with exotic French names on their labels abound, many people still turn to carbonated, sugared, or caffeinated drinks rather than imbibing just pure, clean water.

Wake up call: There are few people who get any benefit from sports drinks. If one eats normal, reasonably nutritious meals, there is no need for extra vitamins, electrolytes or *energy enhancers* just because you've jogged a few miles.

Short of being a professional athlete who spends entire days in heavy physical activity, these hyper-marketed products benefit only the bottom line of the companies that sell them. Healthy individuals have enough nutrients and salts stored in their tissues to get through a solid workout without ill effect. The only thing that should be replaced with intention is the water itself.

Drink pure, clean water.

You eat highly salted foods. An unattractive level of salt is stored in your body. You need to *eliminate* as much of that from your body as possible, and exercise—sweating—is a great way to do it. You don't want to replace all that excess salt. It is likely that there is enough salt in the dressing you will pour over your salad at lunch to replace what you've sweated off.

Choose foods prepared with *sea-salt* rather than table salt. Replace your salt at home with sea-salt. It *salts*, but has a healthier spectrum of minerals and electrolytes. Sea-salt has nutritional value, whereas table salt does not.

Drink pure, clean water.

What about caffeine and those energy boosters? They're just a cheat. They make you feel like you're doing more, but for the amount of stress and harm they do to your endocrine system (adrenal glands, etc.) they do not sufficiently improve fat-burning, cardio-enhancement or muscle building—the purposes for which you're doing exercise.

Drink pure, clean water.

If you're a teen engaged in a four-hour football practice in August in Miami, then adding electrolytes to one's water has some credence, just as soldiers in the South Pacific took salt pills to sustain them while they spent their days digging trenches on far-flung island outposts during World War II.

However, if you're of the age, lifestyle, and situation where reading this book has context, it's just not necessary.

Drink pure, clean water.

What is "pure, clean water?" First, what it's not: It's not tap water. Nor is it distilled water; distillation removes the minerals, and water must have some minerals both for taste and as an added source of these elements. It should not have any of the heavy metals, such as Arsenic, Lead, Mercury, Cadmium, and a host of others.

In 2001, shortly after the new administration took office in Washington, it reversed the initiative of the previous administration and *doubled the allowable amount of Arsenic in drinking water*. There's only one arsenic, and yes, that's the one.

Every indication is that industry has taken advantage of the relaxed restrictions regarding the permissible amount of this poison in our water supply; it's costly to remove and industry saves untold millions of dollars by just leaving it there for you to consume. Water being an important ingredient in cooking, it's in our food as well, inasmuch as Arsenic doesn't boil or cook off. You definitely want to have your water tested if you use it in food preparation.

Special note on Arsenic*:* There are indications that mild arsenic poisoning can directly cause erectile dysfunction by "alteration of the voltage-gated potassium channel" which is a control mechanism of the circulatory system and required for erectile function.

If at all possible, you want to seek an alternate, clean source of water for drinking and cooking; bathing is not an issue. Those large 5-gallon bottles you might see in offices and business that are provided by spring-water companies are a good choice as long as the water actually comes from a clean, spring source. Bottled water that is simply *purified* tap water is not acceptable.

Fluoride and chlorine are poisons that are intentionally added to municipal water systems—your tap water. Let's look at them.

The ability of **fluoride** to prevent cavities was first discovered in the Western US at the beginning of the twentieth century. There was a naturally high concentration of fluoride in the drinking water in several communities in Colorado. While it stained teeth a dark brown, sometimes almost black, it also seemed to convey a barrier to cavities.

There were many other dental issues among the residents of those towns in which this was first observed; fluoride was not—and is not—a panacea of dental health. A rigorous program of education—teaching children proper dental hygiene—was instituted and that created measurable improvements in the teeth of residents in those communities.

However, some genius, having noted and singled out the cavity preventing effect, had an idea: what if fluoride was introduced into the water supplied by municipal systems and distributed to the public without giving them a choice? Might that reduce the occurrence of dental decay?

After a few decades, a program destined to spread nationwide was initiated to do just that, and today few people who draw their water from a utility—as opposed to their own well—escape fluoridation.

Well, it may have prevented tooth decay, but fluoride is a toxin and it messes with many other functions of the body. In the world of 1945, when fluoride was first introduced into the public water supply, it probably did little noticeable harm. Maybe. But in 1945 people weren't subjected to the wide spectrum of chemicals and artificial ingredients in their food all contributing to toxic load.

Further, recent reports have indicated that people are getting too much fluoride. Overdose through the unnatural addition of fluoride to water actually softens teeth doing exactly the opposite of what was intended. This is yet another case of dreadful unintended consequences—a side effect.

> *Fluoride is a poison that disrupts brain activity and assaults every cell of your body and should be avoided completely.*

As far as its intended purpose, proper daily dental care eliminates the need for fluoride in drinking water and in toothpaste. Go fluoride free!

Chlorine, as opposed to fluoride, has no alleged medical benefit. It is used in the purification of municipal water supplies in the same way it is used in swimming pools. It kills bacteria, viruses and other microorganisms. It also kills you.

Cytotoxicity—the ability to poison and kill cells—is not specific to the buggers in the water; chlorine has a deleterious effect on your body cells and your overall well-being. The chemical is an irritant and inflames tissues. Lots more about inflammation later.

So if the water you're drinking brings to mind that wonderful vacation where you lounged poolside for hours, don't drink it! That reminiscence is being triggered by the smell of chlorine that remains in the water after it has left the water treatment plant. It will poison you and slap Harry down.

Water should be free of fluoride, chlorine, heavy metals, bacteria (most commonly those called coliforms) and compounds such as benzene or anything with a name you find difficult to pronounce. Screw the FDA; setting a "limit" on the amount of poisonous chemicals in your water or food is just pandering to the economic desires of big businesses. ***There is no acceptable amount of poison in your food, in your water, or in your body.***

How Much Water?

The most publicized wisdom is that an adult should drink eight, eight-ounce glasses of water each day. That's 64 ounces. That's half a gallon. That's nuts.

Drink when you're thirsty. And drink half of the times when you're feeling hungry. Most hunger, especially when you feel like having a snack after you've consumed a respectable sized meal an hour earlier, is really thirst triggered by excess salt in your food. It is easy for the brain-body to confuse the two.

Watch the color of your pee—it's the very best indicator of the state of your hydration. It should be pale yellow; if it's clear, that's okay. If it appears bright yellow, you need to drink some water. If it's deep yellow, you need to drink a bunch of water, but it's better to space out a few glasses over an hour or two rather than down a huge amount all at once.

And you should pee several times a day. We guys can drain the snake at almost any time and hold-it for much longer than can most women. But if you have no urge to go throughout the day, then you should get some water into you.

By "water," I mean water. Not soda or anything carbonated, or coffee, or the sports drink, or iced or hot tea or anything else that contains water. Drink only pure, clean water.

A Note on Drinking at Meals

Digestion begins in the mouth while you're chewing. Saliva contains important enzymes that chemically break down your food. Further, the physical action of chewing breaks up what you're eating so the digestive juices in your stomach can come into greater contact with what you've swallowed. Digestion improves when you chew your food well.

Water is primarily absorbed from your gut in the large intestine which is the last organ of digestion. The stomach and small intestine precede it.

When you drink a lot of liquid with your meals—habitually taking a sip after every bite—the acids and enzymes that are secreted into your stomach and small intestine to digest your food are diluted. You're hampering digestion. The body tries to compensate by producing more acid and more enzymes.

My personal, *gut* feeling is that a lifetime of this eating-drinking habit may be the source of acid production issues that results in gastroesophageal reflux disease: GERD, or acid reflux.

Try to reduce the amount of liquid—soda, beer, and even water—that you drink as you're eating. If you get very thirsty while you're eating, then your food has too much salt. That's another issue.

Chew well. Reduce fluid intake when eating. When you do drink, drink pure, clean water.

A Two-Way Street

I've discussed the issues of eating badly and how that results in poor digestion as food and drink move through the alimentary canal toward its final disposal. Sometimes things move in the opposite direction.

GERD is yet another vein of gold for the pharmaceutical industry in its never-ending quest to mine your wallet. It's not natural. I'm convinced that while it is a real disease, and can become chronic and possibly irreversible, its basic cause for those forty and up is the decades of poor food, drink and lifestyle choices.

In an initial draft of this book, I wrote the following in reference to acid reflux:

I've got it, too. And no matter how well I eat and drink now— avoiding alcohol, coffee, sodas, and other offenders for an extended period of time—if I don't take my omeprazole every day, the less expensive and fully effective generic of Prilosec OTC®, I'll wake up in the middle of the night with the fires of hell burning in my chest.

I went on to explain that omeprazole is the only drug that I allowed myself inasmuch as it has few side effects for an otherwise healthy individual, none of which I experienced. This is another benefit of a healthier lifestyle. When you do need to take a medication for a disease, infection, or disorder, it will both work more effectively, and do so with fewer, if any, of the possible side-effects. Still, I wasn't happy about taking omeprazole as there's anecdotal evidence that links this drug to ED.

I find that I have to correct myself. Subsequent to that writing, I ran out of omeprazole, and neglected to buy any for several days. I went cold turkey. No acid reflux returned, so I never took it again. That was years ago; with better eating habits, I don't need the medication, something my doctor told me would never happen.

When I wrote my initial observations, I had not given the effects of my healthier lifestyle enough time to reverberate throughout my body. It took years to get me to where I needed the medication. So, experience has shown me, it could take time (in my case, a full year) to repair my digestion, heal my esophageal lining, and make the GERD medication unnecessary.

For those of you who are cost conscious, the money I save by not buying this medication more than pays my Netflix bill each month. A guy's gotta have his priorities.

> ***Special note on GERD***: DO NOT take omeprazole or any medication for GERD without the recommendation of a physician. Not all chronic heartburn is reflux. Taking these drugs when not medically appropriate will do you harm. Worse, you could miss addressing the real cause of your heartburn, something far more serious.

Most of this book is about my personal observations. My experiences seem to be getting better all the time. After years on my new healthier lifestyle, I'm free of all medications. Let me restate that I still do enjoy my scotch—though I drink on a weekly basis not daily—I enjoy fully caffeinated coffee—in the morning not all day long—and I even indulge in the occasional greasy patty-melt with French fries at the diner—emphasis on the word "occasional!"

What improvements in your overall health might you achieve with some patience and willpower? And what unexpected consequences—*positive side effects*—might you enjoy by following some of the guidelines laid down on these pages? Try it. Find out.

Chapter 9: Eating Habits

Vegetarianism

Everyone needs vegetable matter as part of their diet, and vegetable matter alone *can* provide all the protein and other nutritional essentials. But eliminating all meat protein—beef, pork, lamb, chicken, fish, etc.—without intelligently adding a wide variety of vegetarian foods can push you into nutritional deficit.

A Naturopathic doctor once told me that the unhealthiest people she sees in her practice are vegetarians—those people who won't eat meat. They become convinced that meat is bad and they just decide to give it up without any consideration for their personal, quite individual, biochemistry. In most cases, they need some amount of animal protein in their diet. While there are some people who are genetically predisposed to vegetarianism, it's likely you don't want to be one of them.

Vegetarians don't eat meat, but will eat animal products such as eggs and milk. This separates them from Vegans who won't eat meat AND won't eat animal products. Uber-vegans won't wear leather either, creating a religion out of their food choices to the point they dispute the scientific facts that human teeth and digestive systems are eminently evolved to acquire, process, and productively extract nutrition from animals and their byproducts. Animals eat animals. We are animals. Veganism is technically unnatural for humans, but then again, so is reading.

There are few people who can successfully be vegetarians and that has as much to do with societal pressures as personal constitution. Fewer can survive as vegans. If good health, fitness, muscle mass, stamina, and skin tone—this last being a huge barometer for a positive state of health—is attained while an individual enjoys a vegetarian or vegan lifestyle, I am not one to cast aspersions.

It takes a lot of work, not necessarily to *be* a vegetarian or vegan, but to *become* one; the transition takes effort. Try it and prove me wrong. Most of the work has to do with functioning in a Western culture surrounded by delectable dishes, most of which include meat, poultry, or fish.

It is well documented, through *The China Study* as well as other clinical investigations, that the Western diet includes too much meat. Beef, pork, chicken or turkey, fish. In that order. Health, especially in the arena of reducing cancer rates, coincides with a reduction in animal protein. But even the originator of that study, a proponent of a meat-free diet, found that a complete elimination of meat is not necessary; fifteen percent or less meat in the diet has little harmful effect.

What the Western diet does wrong is invert the proportions of the food groups. Most of our food should be vegetable based, and meat should be a small addition. We generally do the opposite.

Throughout this presentation, I'm taking into consideration the audience—men—and the mindset of Americans and those worldwide who have become Americanized in their eating habits. I make no insistence on swinging the pendulum too far.

Consider meeting half way. Cut down on meat. If not at a single meal, then on one's daily load. You're reading this book because you have a problem. Three meat-meals a day is a Harry-killer.

This is a guide that is meant to be *practical* above all else. As a discussion aimed at men, vegetarianism isn't an issue. But I will promote the idea that many of us should *cut down* on the amount of meat and increase the vegetable component of our daily diets.

Balance is the key. There is no precise formula for the proportions of meat, carbs, vegetables, fruits, and starches that an individual should strive to achieve; everyone is different. The old food pyramid concocted by the Food and Drug Administration was a wild-assed guess. Everyone has to create their own pyramid.

Food Combination

And here's our next challenge. Food combining is an essential part of a dick-healthy diet. More precisely, it's a matter of understanding which foods should *not* be combined, that is, not eaten at the same meal.

The beauty is you don't have to give up anything. You just have to eat them at separate times.

The demonstrable fact is that having a large glass of milk with that big steak or slab of roast beef, guarantees digestive issues. These first manifest as, "What crawled up your ass and died?" Later on, they turn into other dangerous maladies (that's a hint).

Meat and milk are digested in different ways. Milk—and all dairy products—interfere with the proper and complete digestion of meat, especially in the essential primary breakdown processes that occur in the stomach. This causes meat protein to be insufficiently prepared for further digestion as it enters the small intestine. Think of what quickly happens to a car's engine if gasoline, oil and air are not properly filtered before they enter an engine.

Once meat that has not been properly digested in the stomach enters the small intestine, anaerobic bacteria—the predominant bugs in the intestines—go to town turning out all manner of chemical compounds that are similar to those found in the foul smelling sludge at the bottom of a swamp. These substances not only smell terrible, but they are toxic. These chemicals are absorbed into your blood stream and spread throughout your body.

The harm these toxins do doesn't become apparent until decades later causing the phenomenon we call "getting old."

Regarding Milk

Humans are the only animals that drink milk after being weaned from the teat. All other animals seek out vegetation, or eat other animals, or some combination of the two, and never go back to milk.

Human ingenuity and technology has introduced milk into our diets in spite of the fact that it is a largely foreign substance from another genus of animal.

In some less industrialized cultures, milk is very necessary as a source of vitamins and calories. However, these peoples do not live with the overall toxic stress of the Western lifestyle. Americans, however, have gone completely over the top with the mythology that children need milk to grow strong bones... blah, blah, blah... you've all heard the marketing nonsense spewed out by the multi-billion dollar dairy industry.

My daughter—breast fed until just before her first birthday, and twenty years old as of this writing—never had animal milk until she was four years old. A friend's mother gave her a glass at their home. Since then she has had a glass of milk less often than once a month, again when outside our home. Yes, she has some cheese and certainly ice cream—in moderation. But her digestive tract was not, and is not, bathed in dairy on a daily basis. As a result, she has never had sinus or ear problems, does not have allergies. She is rarely sick. She's slim and has good skin tone. She still consumes milk products infrequently—a minor fraction of what most average Americans take in.

How is this possible? How can she have any bones at all? According to the dairy industry, milk is essential to a child's growth! Simple, there are lots of other foods that are high—often higher—in calcium and all the other important nutrients touted as found in milk. These foods, however, do not have the unhealthy quantities of fat and sugar that is a major constituent of milk. Additionally, by feeding her cruciferous vegetables—those naturally high in calcium, such as broccoli—instead of milk and dairy products, my daughter has not been subjected to the enormous hormone and antibiotic load that taints milk and has been postulated to lead to breast cancer later in life.

Peoples who society depend on dairy for a major portion of their nutrition, generally milk their own livestock and drink raw milk that is free from added hormones, antibiotics, and pasteurization. Further, they do not drink it with meat.

You may want to watch an interview with *Robert Cohen* or visit the *Not Milk* website. Web addresses are provided at the end of this book.

An aside:

The Dairy-Industrial-Complex injects female hormones into cows that cause them to produce more milk. These hormones are passed along in the milk to those who drink it. I often wonder if those mammary production enhancers might upset the normal hormone balance of brawny men who like an ice-cold glass of milk with their roast beef sandwich. Could those girly hormones accumulate in their macho bodies and begin to take their toll later in life? Could Harry be getting in touch with his feminine side when he refuses to perform? It's just a thought.

There is no nutritional need to ever drink milk. You can survive—especially if you eat meat—without ever having any dairy whatsoever… ever. And with the evidence that milk is a cancer promoter, you'd be much better off keeping dairy consumption to an absolute minimum. Cut it out if you can.

15% Meat: What Does that Mean?

I cited researchers (T. Colin Campbell, *The China Study*) who have determined that as much as 15% of one's diet can be meat with little health effect. Okay. 15% of what? Of the weight? Of the square inches of the dinner plate?

The answer is calories. The percentages that are specified are always relative to the calorie content of the food. If one was to consume 1,000 calories at a meal, then 15% = 150 calories could come from meat.

But how do you calculate that without precise measurements of the weight of food and an intimate knowledge of the calories per ounce (or gram) of every ingredient in a prepared meal? You can't. Further, does this need to apply to every meal? What if you're "off" one meal? Do you adjust the next meal? What if you have to wait two meals to make up the difference? It's entirely unworkable.

To start improving your nutrition to regain potency and achieve some modicum of health and vitality so you can enjoy healthy sex for life, you need to use common sense.

You know how much meat you eat now. Two burgers and a hot dog at the barbeque? Cut out one burger. Bada-bing, you've cut your meat consumption almost in half. Force yourself to eat a small salad at meals and give some of your French fries to the dog. Leave the cheese off your burger—you probably can't taste it anyway—and you've cut out some calories and the harmful effects of hormone-laden dairy. It's not portion control, it's *selective* portion control; you can still eat as much vegetables, fruits, and melons as you'd like.

Oh, and eat a freaking apple (or pear, plum, peach) once a day. Once you've grown accustomed to having one piece of fruit a day, up it to two or three. It will stabilize blood sugar, cut down the mid-day munchies, and eliminate the 3:00PM wall, so you can stop taking energy drinks that kill you pecker and make you fat.

That's how you up your vegetable intake and reduce meat, adjust percentages and proportions, and move toward a balanced, boner-friendly diet. How far you take it over time is your choice. You'll likely feel better just by cutting down on the harshest offenders. If you have major health problems in addition to ED, you'll be best served by reducing the amount of meat you eat to a sustainable minimum, and upping all the categories of vegetarian foods: fruits, vegetables, nuts, seeds, berries, legumes, etc.

Read my book, "Lose Weight with Nutritional Leverage," for a suggested way to regain vitality and longevity. It's less about losing weight and more about gaining health through nutrition—including erectile health.

Chapter 10: Inflammation Nation

At some point in your life you've had an infection at the site of an abrasion or cut. It gets painful—inflamed. The redness is a sign that your immune system is protecting tissues that are under attack by bacteria or viruses. Inflammation is also part of the healing process.

Whether it's the back of your throat, the scraped skin on your knee, the iridescent area of your sunburned shoulders, the allergic reaction surrounding a mosquito bite, *or the irritation of the blood vessels throughout your body*, the basic bodily defense mechanism is the same. At the microscopic level, immune cells move to the injury and proliferate. Lymph fills the area; it swells. Any dangerous microbes that have entered through the wound are attacked. Damaged and dead cells are isolated and removed. The healing process begins.

Or does it? What happens when you keep bumping that sore on your hand? If you keep bumping your hand, the soreness stays and might even spread until you take care to protect it with a bandage.

If your eyes are irritated, they get red and itchy. When your sinuses are under attack, you get a runny nose or your head fills up and your nasal passages are blocked. These are signs, and because they're so annoying you'll take some action to address them. You may take an antihistamine, but that doesn't cure you, it just covers up the symptoms. Or, you may get a HEPA-filter for your home, and eliminate the irritants from your environment.

But what happens if the nerves and blood vessels that control erection are inflamed? Until now, you didn't know that's what's killing your dick. Will you take some action? You can pop the expensive pills or you can address the root cause. And that root cause—as is often the case in many diseases—is systemic inflammation, an immune response most often to food.

Because we all bathe ourselves in foods to which we are allergic—yes, you do—we are all in a constant state of sub-clinical inflammation. It is termed *sub-clinical*, because the allergy doesn't express itself as demonstrably as itchy eyes, stuffed sinuses, or a bright red rash.

We call it "sub-clinical" because we don't feel "sick," or do we?

If your sinuses are congested, or you sneeze and cough in the absence of any noticeable irritant, or you don't feel well after a meal because you are bloated, or your farts smell like road-kill, then you know that you have a problem. Your doctor may not be able to diagnose your issues, but that doesn't mean you don't have something wrong. By definition, your dis-ease is sub-clinical—less than clinical—but must not be ignored.

Have you ever heard of someone that had *never been sick in his life*, and was diagnosed with cancer? Never been sick in his life? He's been sick for many years. He just didn't know it because it was—for the umpteenth time—SUB-CLINICAL! It didn't give him any overt signs.

There's a parable that's been floating around on the Internet for a number of years. I retell it here, in the shortest possible iteration, for the benefit of those few people who may not have encountered it:

There's a pious preacher who lives in a town being threatened by a flood. *(Remember the story yet?)* A neighbor comes by in a pickup truck and calls to him, "The flood is coming. Get in my truck." The preacher says, "No, thank you. The Lord will provide." The waters start to rise. Some other people come by in a small boat and offer him safe evacuation. "No thank you," he repeats. "The Lord will provide." Finally, he's standing on his roof as the water climbs to record levels. A police helicopter hovers over him and offers him escape. Again, "No, thank you. The Lord will provide." As his house is consumed by the flood and he's about to be swept away, he calls to heaven, "Lord, why have you forgotten me?" The clouds rumble and a voice says, "Forgotten you? I sent you a truck, a boat, and a helicopter."

The person who, until his dooming diagnosis, claims never to have been sick in his life, is a person who has never given heed to all the signs of disease right up to the point that it's impossible to ignore. "It's just allergies," they'll say in the presence of a cold that just won't go away. "Musta et somethin' bad," they say to explain stomach, digestive, or bowel issues that recur frequently. And then there's the perennial, "I'm just feeling tired today." This mantra may be repeated frequently day after day for years. It is not normal to always be tired. Lack of energy, lethargy, or the inability to stay awake throughout the day is a sign of more significant issues. And erectile dysfunction is a symptom, too.

Chronic Fatigue Syndrome (CFS)

A *syndrome* is a term used by the medical community to lump together a number of symptoms that tend to occur at the same time. The idea is to alert physicians to a possible state of disease. A syndrome is not same as a disease; it is a collection of symptoms that exists when no disease can be identified as causing the symptoms. Basically, it's an "I don't know" on the part of the medical establishment. It's codified bullshit.

CFS is a syndrome because they don't know what causes it, though some researchers believe it is an inflammation of the nervous system due to some unknown causative agent. Sound familiar? The syndrome occurs most often in women ages thirty to fifty. I'm guessing it's because so many men are in just such shitty shape as they approach forty that CFS is masked by everything else that's wrong with them.

This is a classic example of how a cutting-edge, state of the art medical machine, as we have in pure and applied research, can completely overlook the obvious. Most people are in a state of systemic—whole body—inflammation all the time. For some it rises to the point of a clinical "syndrome."

For other, perhaps, their dicks stop working, and there's a pill for that, so it's no big deal, right? Wrong.

Not being able to get or sustain an erection is a symptom of other processes going on in the body and should not be ignored. Just because you don't have anybody with whom to "do it," don't think that it doesn't matter. It matters.

When you do find someone, dealing with it by popping an ED pill that you get from a friend or an Internet drug store—in the absence of a medical examination—is playing Russian roulette with your life. Get it checked out. When your doctor tells you that it's just part of getting older, congratulations, you don't have one of the labeled diseases.

Breathe a sigh of relief, then, appreciate what I'm presenting to you in these pages. It's not a sign of getting older. It's a sign of getting unhealthier and it will catch up to you in other ways, too.

> *My hypothesis is that erectile dysfunction may be yet another manifestation of whole-body, sub-clinical inflammation due to allergic reactions to food, drink, as well as exposure to environmental factors—household pets, for example—that set off a cascade of immune responses within the body.*

I say "another manifestation" to make it clear that I am adding ED to the list of those outward signs of reaction that are more generally accepted as allergies, just as sinus and breathing issues, watery eyes, and fluid retention are so often diagnosed.

Nitric Oxide—Part II

> *The inflammatory process chews up nitric oxide, reducing the quantity available to produce an erection.*

Depending on the severity of your sub-clinical inflammation, this essential compound may be reduced in concentration below the levels necessary for any performance whatsoever.

Inflammation, all by itself, is anti-erectile. Inflammation can be burning up your love-life.

There are ways to increase nitric oxide concentrations, within safe levels, for the promotion of penile erection. It has to be done naturally and with gentle finesse.

Should you consider an ED drug—hopefully just as a stopgap—make sure you discuss their use with your doctor. There's a reason these are prescription drugs.

Smoking

Smoking irritates and inflames body tissues and decreases the amount of nitric oxide in the body. It will exaggerate the effects of other erectile deterrents… 'nough said.

How to Put Out the Flames

So what can you do to reduce or eliminate chronic sub-clinical inflammation that is affecting your overall health and contributes to your ED?

Your response to your situation can range from mild adjustments in your diet to an all-out crusade to reclaim your erectile muse—your wood nymph, as it were.

First, a reality check: when someone eats something to which they are specifically allergic, they have a reaction—mild or severe. The reaction dissipates over time and is gone when the allergen, the substance that caused the reaction, is out of their system.

This does not hold true for sub-clinical, whole-body inflammation. A course of action that cleans and clears the body of the offending substances—plural—must be pursued. The buzz-word is "Detox," short for detoxification. There are many plans available from many vendors and each health practitioner has one they prefer. Some work very well. Others are a sham.

The best detox is the slow, purification achieved by eating right and allowing your body to cleanse itself. It takes longer, but you will avoid the *healing crisis* that is common to detox programs. This is a period when you feel like shit, but your health practitioner says you're supposed to. It's analogous to those first critical days of cleansing by drug abusers, though not anywhere as severe and doesn't require medical supervision.

I've stated that erectile dysfunction is the aggregate effect of the factors I've discussed so far, plus others I will enumerate later. When it comes to inflammation, it's the overwhelming assault of all the foods, drinks, and lifestyle factors that irritate internal body tissues.

The Perfect World

In a perfect world where we all had absolute willpower, here's how you'd approach your problem. It's the same as if you were trying to find the cause of a life threatening allergic reaction.

Remember, this is just a mental exercise, not something I'm suggesting.

• Eliminate all food and drink, stripping your intake down to a minimum number of different foods to which you know you're not allergic, and eliminate all foods that are known to be highly allergenic: nuts, shellfish, etc. Eat only those foods that are generally known to not produce allergies: non-berry vegetables, fruit, beef.

• Eat only these limited foods, and drink pure, clean water for two weeks, or until your allergic reactions completely disappear. In the case of general allergies, this would be the elimination of sneezing, coughing, lung irritation, skin eruptions, etc.

Let's presume that this single, albeit draconian dietary adjustment works. Your outward allergies disappear, and you feel your performance coming back.

• You then start adding a few—just a few—of the foods you previously enjoyed back into your diet. Wait a few days, and see that you're not affected.

• In reality, sneezing, congestion, skin irritation, etc. will manifest much earlier and quicker than the effects on your pecker. So if you start getting those reactions, you will want to note what foods may have caused your irritation. Those foods most recently reintroduced to your diet include an offender. Take those off your diet. Otherwise, over time, you may notice some effect on Harry's performance, too.

• Add other foods back. Repeat until you have identified all the foods to which you are allergic and don't eat them again.

But this is not a perfect world and few of us have the self-control to suffer through this regimen. There's an easier way.

While I'm going to approach a course of action in terms of an aggressive overall health campaign, I'm not going to suggest anything that is not doable.

As a start, eliminate those foods and drinks that directly affect you; those foods to which you KNOW that you have an allergy.

Don't say, "It only gives me a little gas, so I'll only have a little and take an anti-gas pill." The gas is a symptom. You can't excuse a food which "...makes me itchy, so I'll take an antihistamine." The itch is a symptom. Drugs just cover it up on the outside, but you're still assaulting your man-machine on the inside. These things must be completely removed from your diet.

Next, eliminate or reduce your intake of those things that inflame everyone's tissues.

Universal Causes of Inflammation

Very high on the list are carbonated drinks. Few of you will be willing to eliminate sodas and other carbonated soft drinks, but cutting down on them is essential. Here's why: You may remember some of this from high school chemistry class.

pH is a measure of how acid or alkaline a liquid is. pH 7.0 is neutral, pH's below 7.0 are acidic, and above 7.0 are alkaline.

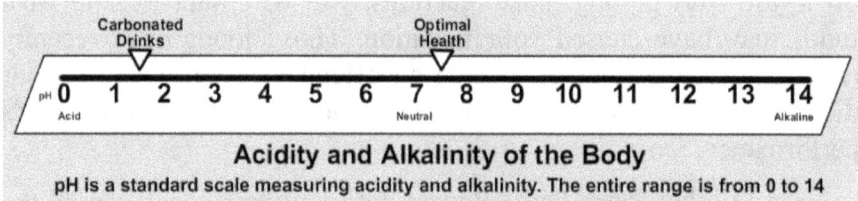

Acidity and Alkalinity of the Body
pH is a standard scale measuring acidity and alkalinity. The entire range is from 0 to 14

The human body functions optimally at a slightly alkaline pH, about 7.4 or 7.5. Cancers don't grow well in an alkaline environment, so, all by itself that should provide some incentive to raise your pH, that is, alkalize your body.

Carbonated water is carbolic acid, and has a pH of 1. Carbonated drinks have a pH of between 1 and 2. While your body has a sophisticated buffering system, that is, it can neutralize and "absorb" a lot of acid without suffering immediate effects, if you bathe your innards with your favorite non-alcoholic bubbly and double-down with high caffeine content—caffeine is also an acid—you are acidifying your body.

What you eat and drink can rapidly drop the pH of your body to below 6. By metabolic standards, that's very acidic. When you've lived a carbonated lifestyle for twenty, thirty, or forty years, your blood vessels have been subjected to an environment that promotes inflammation, disease, aging, and a limp dick.

Blood vessels, as the primary producer of nitric oxide will all but shut down production when inflamed. Besides ED, every other cardio-vascular catastrophe waits in the wings.

Coffee, Tea, and Other Caffeinated Drinks

Have a cup or two to start the day, but don't drown your insides by pounding it down all day long. As far as Harry is concerned, energy drinks are pure poison. Eliminate these entirely. If you feel you must get your caffeine boost because you've *hit the wall* in the afternoon, all by itself, that's a sign of poor nutrition, bad food combination, or an allergic reaction to something you've eaten.

Hitting the 3:00PM wall is a sign of poor nutrition. Afternoon fatigue is a symptom; it is not normal for a healthy individual that has gotten a regular night's sleep. Flip-side: sleeplessness, or the inability to awake rested, is yet another symptom of poor nutrition and bad food combination.

Too much caffeine will acidify your body, directly irritate nerves and blood vessels, and add to the toxic load to which you're exposing Harry.

Drink citrus juices in moderation. In addition to being very acid, they aid in leaching calcium from the body and erode the enamel on your teeth. Though, that's an entirely different story.

But how can you live without a soda with your hamburger at the park? Can you really just stop drinking coffee? Nope. Don't even try. But you can cut down. I'll be discussing how much of these poisons your body can accommodate—the dose response—later on.

Reminder: ***It is the cumulative effect of all the things you do to offend and disrupt your metabolism that negatively impacts your overall health and has a direct impact on potency.***

Avoid diet sodas, or diet anything for that matter. Aspartame (the most commonly used artificial sweetener), is toxic and causes whole-body inflammation. Google "Dr. Russell Blaylock aspartame" to watch an informative video. And beware of "amino sweet," the new name for aspartame approved by the FDA to deceive you into thinking it's safe.

Diet sodas offend your body in two ways. First, by making your body more acidic, and second, by introducing a toxin that attacks nerve cells in the brain and elsewhere. Plus: aspartame laced drinks do not help you lose or control your weight, they do just the opposite, leading to hyperinsulinism, stressing the adrenal glands, and greatly increases the likelihood that you'll have ED—that makes it a *triple whammy*.

I shudder even to type these words, but you should cut down on alcohol, but you don't need to stop drinking completely.

Joke Time: W. C. Fields once said, "I feel sorry for anyone who doesn't drink. When they get up in the morning, that's as good as they're going to feel all day."

There's some wisdom that punches through this humor, and I'll be addressing that just a few chapters hence. But, if you don't drink alcohol, that's okay. It's just a joke. I'm not proselytizing for alcohol consumption.

Alcohol inflames tissues including, but not limited to, your blood vessels. While red wine has been touted as healthy, it is generally accepted that one doesn't drink an entire bottle at a sitting. A glass or two is optimal. Which doesn't mean that occasional transgression is going to shut Harry down completely—I'm not promoting it, I just live in the real world. There is a time-response as well as a dose-response to drinking. If getting drunk is limited to March 17th each year, you shouldn't have health problems.

If you drink hard liquor or beer excessively every day, the constant irritation of your vessels and tissues can accumulate over time and contribute to your ED.

Alcohol slows the response to stimulation even in young men who are normally quick to arousal (remember?). It also deadens touch-nerves so you won't feel the sensation of her efforts to get you ready for the deed.

I'm not suggesting that you not have a before-dinner drink, or that you shouldn't enjoy wine with the entree. But you may want to skip the after-dinner libation if you expect to get your freak-on later that night... whether or not you're employing an ED medication.

The immediate application of alcohol before sex is anti-erectile. The long-term use of excessive quantities of alcohol may cause all-out erectile dysfunction.

Chapter 11: The Dose Makes the Poison

In the 16th century, Paracelsus, a Renaissance physician said, "All things are poison and nothing is without poison, only the dose permits something not to be poisonous." In some academic and medical circles, his observations and conclusions have earned him the title of "the father of modern toxicology."

By "...dose permits something not to be poisonous," he means—as has been borne out by modern medicine—that in small enough quantities, the body can assimilate, accommodate, or eliminate many substances including those that are categorized as poisons. Sure there are exceptions like manufactured nerve agents, but that's not what we're discussing here.

We know the converse of Paracelcus' statement also to be true. A thing that is generally considered entirely safe to eat or drink can be made lethal by consuming extraordinary quantities: a few beers, a couple of glasses of wine, or several shots of liquor can be festive; in extraordinary quantities, however, alcohol can kill.

But it's the dose-response to substances that attack our health that bring us to…

The Nexus of My Hypothesis

The effects are cumulative; the quantity of each individual toxic substance may be small, but the effect of all these substances adds up and puts you past the event horizon; they'll ruin your health and kill your dick.

Remember when I warned you that ED could be the symptom of a much more dangerous disease in your body? Even if you doctor doesn't find anything overtly wrong, as my doctor didn't find in me, know that erectile dysfunction is an indicator of a general lack of health that will lead to any number of disabilities later on. High blood pressure and high cholesterol are not diseases of the aged.

They're diseases brought about by decades of being unhealthy, not just by the decades. Head the warning.

- It's not just that aspartame in your diet drinks is inflaming your tissues, and
- It's not just that fluffy the cat's dander is producing allergic reactions in your body, and
- It's not just that you eat high animal, low vegetable meals, and
- It's not just bad combinations of foods such as milk and meat, and
- It's not just the alcohol consumption, and
- It's not just the acidification of our bodies, and
- It's not just the high-stress lifestyle…
- *…It's ALL OF IT added together!*

When you treat yourself like a septic tank and pour shit into yourself every day, at some point, years down the road, you're going to overflow. You'll have to be pumped out, and that will include cardiac bypass surgery, bowel resection, prostate removal, walkers and wheelchairs, and a fist full of pills every day for the remainder of an unhealthy, uncomfortable, celibate life.

You never know when you've had sex for the last time, so do all you can to make it in your eighties, not your sixties or earlier. But if you're already there, if you're already on medications and have health issues besides the ED, know that much is reversible—the exception being the replacement of organs already removed.

Unless you're a member of an isolated tribe deep in the Amazon forest, as you age, your arteries will harden from the accumulated assaults of low levels of these substances. This loss of elasticity naturally effects erectile function. The healthiest member of Western industrialized society, just from living, breathing our air, drinking our water and participating in our stressful lifestyle, will lose some potency as years progress. There is no evolutionary protection against this. We're not supposed to live into our sixties, seventies, and beyond, and we're certainly not supposed to be sexually active as long as we'd like to be.

However, loss of some potency—you won't be able to hammer a 10-penny nail through a mahogany board as in your youth—and reduction in frequency—you may have to skip the double-header at lunch—is normal and shouldn't affect an adult relationship.

When we overdose on inflammatory foods and drinks, and expose ourselves to systemic irritants *and* we do so over long periods of time we affect our bodies in ways that often lead us to the emergency room. Our bodies send us messages that we should not ignore, including the allegorical truck, boat, and helicopter.

ED is the unnecessary shutdown of an entire bodily function— reproduction—that is not a natural lifecycle change in men as menopause is for women (which does not necessarily impact sexuality in the ladies).

ED is a dysfunction that renders you incapable of one of life's most divine pleasures.

ED is reversible, as I've demonstrated for myself, and I hope that what I've presented to you so far will help you begin to work your way through the maze.

But there's a lot more. The treatise continues...

Good News—Bad News

The good news is that, most likely, your ED is reversible.

The bad news is that you can't give up just one thing; it's not a single aspect of your bad diet or lifestyle that's causing your ED, it's a little bit of everything. There will be no "Silver Bullet."

The good news is that you shouldn't have to give up anything completely.

The bad news is that you'll probably have to cut down on many things to some extent.

The good news is that you will have the ultimate feedback-reward mechanism for addressing your issues through diet and lifestyle, in the form of more and better sex.

The bad news is that some of what you have to give up is directly associated with those activities that normally lead to sex, such as a fabulous unhealthy dinner with a bottle of wine followed by a cigar and brandy... or is that Brandie?

The good news is that there is a time-response along with the dose response. It's the effect of dousing your body with chemicals over time, not a single wild night, weekend, or week-long vacation that causes a critical rise in inflammation shutting Harry down.

The bad news is that our human nature tends to forget our long-term objectives. We quickly fall back into old habits after we get home from the vacation, and Harry may go away again.

And finally, the good news is that if you fall off the wagon and start having ED issues, you can once again reverse the process, address your consumption and exercise regimen and get back in the saddle.

The bad news is that each time you cycle around, you're stressing your body even more, causing additional hardening of all your arteries and putting wear-and-tear on all your organs and aging yourself. Fitness should be—must be—a straight and level path.

Chapter 12: Are You Poisoning Harry?

I've discussed food and water, and how many of the things we eat directly or indirectly inflame tissues by immune responses we clump together under an umbrella called *allergies*.

Inflammation of the blood vessels leading to and from the penis, and irritation of the nerves that control erectile response is of primary importance in this discussion.

How do these things make their way to Harry? What can we do to reduce their effect, or minimize their impact to a level below which they might no longer cause dysfunction?

The first place to look is to the fluids that bathe our organs and cells.

Have a Period, Please

Why do most men die before their wives? The old joke says, "Because they want to."

I am sure there are many theories, including simple sex-linked genetic predisposition. However, there's one idea that has been bandied about for many years. It's about blood.

The heart, you know, pumps blood throughout the body. When blood moves through the lungs, it picks up oxygen and delivers it to organs, tissues, and cells from head to toe. Blood collects carbon dioxide, which is poisonous, and discharges it at the lungs.

Nutrition is collected by the intestines and passed to the circulatory system. The nutrients are transported to cells by blood. When cells use the nutrition, it processes it through a series of biochemical reactions, producing energy and the building blocks for tissue growth and repair. But at the end of those reactions, the compounds that are left over are also poisons. *Many of these chemicals are downright deadly.* These are collected by the blood and moved through the liver, which cleans up some, and moves much of it back to the intestines for discharge. Other poisons are filtered by the kidneys and peed away.

This is an overly simplistic presentation. There are many steps that have been omitted for the sake of a quick-and-dirty overview, but here's the take-away:

• The normal process of living produces dangerous chemicals in your body that will kill you, even if you are doing everything perfectly right.

• The liver protects you by chewing up and disposing of some of the bad chemicals, and the kidneys filter out what's left. You eliminate many of these harmful chemicals when you poop and pee.

• And this information matters to you because *the process is not perfect.*

Some of these harmful compounds remain behind. Even in a healthy body, they get circulated in the blood longer than they should. In bodies subjected to the Western diet, livers are overworked and just can't handle the load. These poisons get into tissues via the lymphatic system. They damage cells. Among these poisons are the infamous oxidizing compounds which cause aging, and promote any number of degenerative diseases, including cancer. To battle the oxidizing compounds, we are told by nutritionists to eat foods high in *antioxidants* which neutralize these substances and protect our bodies. Rarely do we hear a nutritionist tell us how to keep oxidants to a minimum in the first place. Avoiding gluten and sugar is a start.

Additionally, there are other chemicals that circulate in our blood that cause harm. They are destroyed and eliminated more slowly. Simply, they sometimes stay for quite a while—long enough to do damage.

Back to the question: why do women live longer than men? One hypothesis has to do with menstruation, that is, a woman's monthly period. Beginning in youth, and lasting about forty years, a woman discharges some blood every month during her period. It's not a lot, but enough—it is thought—to eliminate some of the circulating and hard to eliminate poisons from her circulation. After each menstruation, a woman's blood is replenished; new blood cells are created and fresh plasma is produced. The new blood dilutes the concentration of harmful chemicals, oxidants, free radicals, and other poisons, including some heavy metals that have collected in her blood.

Men don't enjoy this natural bloodletting that may extend life. Even if only a few years, it's significant enough to appear on actuarial charts and affect insurance rates.

How do men catch up? Simple: donate blood. Giving one pint from your system, of the ten to twelve pints in your body, eliminates eight to ten percent of the harmful substances. Within twenty-four hours blood volume is back to normal, and new vibrant red blood cells are replenished within five or six weeks. The rules say that after sixty days you're welcome to donate once more.

Nobody knows if blood donation does what I'm proposing. Does the theory hold any credence whatsoever? Sure. Do doctors agree? Perhaps some few do. Does the FDA support this idea; do they encourage blood donations for this purpose? Nope. Does it hurt to try? Absolutely not!

Supported by the knowledge that blood donation also contributes to the welfare of people in your community, it's an experiment worth performing. Perhaps you are saving a child that has been injured in an automobile accident or a woman fighting for her life after a difficult childbirth, or just lending a hand to some dude that got sloppy with a chainsaw, donation of blood is a kind, generous, and civic-minded activity.

If there's any chance that the idea of the "male period" might prolong your life, why not give it a shot and see if you can live longer? Even if you're on a perfect diet, you're going to accumulate circulating toxins in your blood which include metabolic byproducts that build up and circulate throughout your body, biochemically contributing to the inhibition of erectile function.

Simplified: Blood donation may help you to stop poisoning your dick.

Lymphomania

Okay, we've discussed blood and how it moves nutrients around the body and picks up the poisons that might affect your performance. Blood distributes nutrients throughout the body, but it also passes it off to lymph. It is lymph which bathes every cell and actually delivers the nutrients. In reverse, lymph picks up the waste products of cellular metabolism and takes it back to the blood which transports it to the liver, kidneys, etc.

Lymph is the clear fluid that collects in water blisters. Lymph is the workhorse of cleansing the body of toxic substances that accumulate as part of just being alive. The problem is that lymph doesn't have a pump like the heart that moves it around the body.

The lymphatic system is a network of vessels, similar to veins and arteries, but separate. The actions of your muscles compress and release the lymphatic vessels which have tiny one-way valves inside of them. When you use your muscles, they are squeezed and lymph is moved in one direction only. When your muscles release the vessel, it fills up by suctioning lymph from the segments of the vessels that are upstream. In this way lymph is circulated.

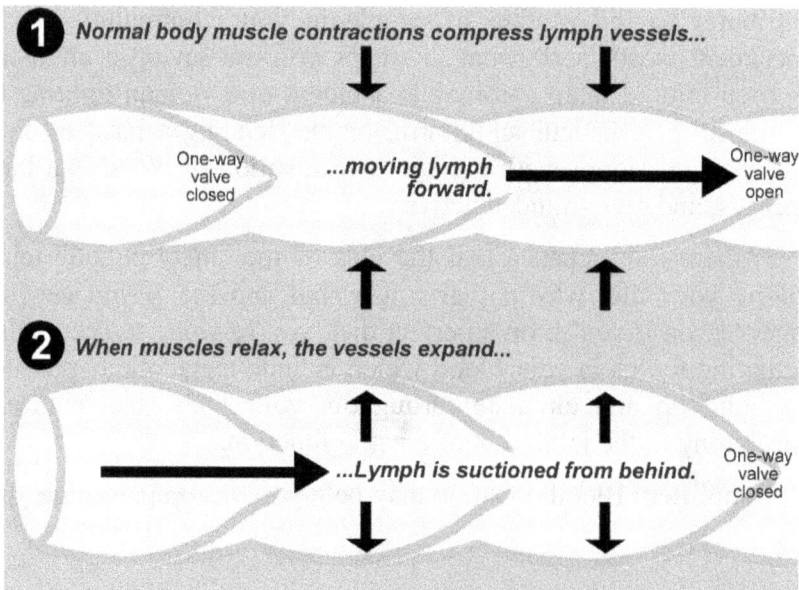

1 Normal body muscle contractions compress lymph vessels...

One-way valve closed

...moving lymph forward.

One-way valve open

2 When muscles relax, the vessels expand...

...Lymph is suctioned from behind.

One-way valve closed

In addition to delivering oxygen and nutrition to cells and removing waste and carbon dioxide, lymph *nodes* are essential to the function of your immune system. Lymphocytes—white blood cells—attack bacteria, viruses, and other pathogens during an infection, then depot the debris at lymph nodes. We are invaded by bacteria and viruses all the time. Lymphocytes and other circulating defender cells of the immune system are on constant alert for microbes and other rogues, such as cancer cells that spring up regularly. A healthy immune system eliminates them quickly. The byproducts of all this housecleaning are toxic and must be shipped off to waste disposal.

The key is that *waste disposal* is accomplished via the blood stream. Lymph has to move to where it can come into intimate contact with blood vessels to pass off the poisons and other leftovers of immunologic function. In the previous section we discussed getting rid of some of the difficult to eliminate substances that linger in our circulatory system, but it is lymph that has those toxins first. We have to clean our lymph, too, but there is no way to siphon off a pint.

To keep lymph moving, you have to move. This goes back to my initial observation that the men depicted in advertising as suffering from ED seem too physically fit to be likely candidates. If an objective poll could be taken, we'd find that most men with ED tend to be largely inactive.

This may not be a sign of slothfulness; it may be occupational. Many of us are confined to cubicles or otherwise chair-ridden as part of our daily routine. Even being on one's feet all day does not provide sufficient exercise to move lymph upwards from the lower extremities of the body. This is the focal point—why I believe that lymph circulation is essential to erectile health.

Lymph nodes—the major collection sites of the lymphatic system—are clustered in a few parts of the body: in the head, around the upper torso and down under your arms, and, most important to our discussion, in the groin, like a glorious halo around you-know-who.

According to my hypothesis, cytotoxic poisons collected by and accumulating in lymph, and perhaps increased hydrostatic lymphatic pressure—gravity acting on accumulated lymph in the lower body—have a deleterious effect on the blood vessels and nerves that are responsible for initiating and maintaining an erection. These impediments, when added to other factors, bring about ED.

So what do you do?

I've designed a simple exercise that can help stimulate that part of lymphatic circulation that is most germane to ED—emptying your lower body of lymphatic sludge. It also stimulates blood flow, increasing nitric oxide production in those areas of the body where it is most essential.

As always, consult your doctor to make sure you're healthy enough to do this exercise. If you have a lower spine injury or are in the throes of any back issue, you may want to defer this until you get an okay from your chiropractor, orthopedist, or physician.

Use common sense, please.

Air Cycling: an Exercise for ED

1. Lie flat on your back in bed. You want to take care not to bruise your spine by lying on a hard surface, so if you use the floor, make sure it is well cushioned.

2. If your stomach muscles—the abdominals—are in sufficient shape to lift both legs at the same time, then you can do both legs simultaneously, bracing yourself with your hands and arms. However, few of us who really need this exercise are in sufficient shape to start with both legs, so I will continue detailing the procedure for those who will raise just one leg at a time.

3. Raise your thigh to about a 90 degree angle with the bed. Keep the other leg bent with foot-down on the bed for leverage.

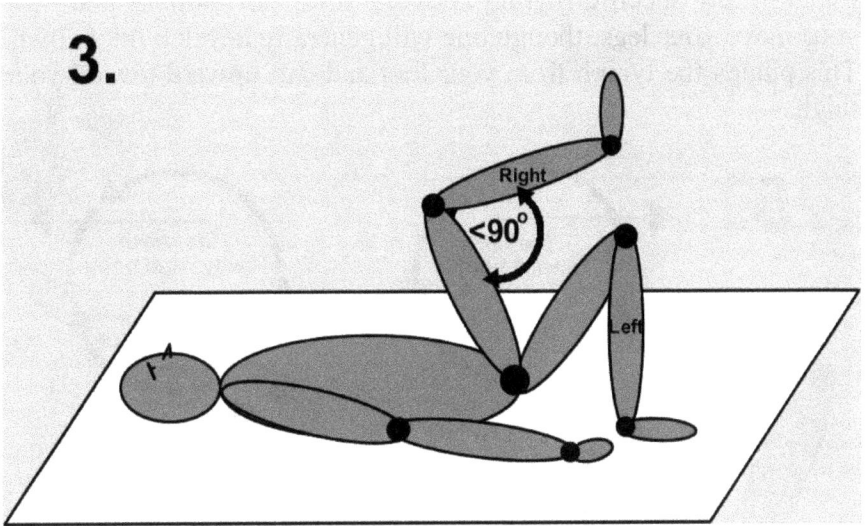

4. Move your foot in an open circle in the air; a bicycle pedaling motion above you. Make a large circle; your leg—thigh relative to calf—should move between a little less than a 90 degree angle to almost, but not quite, straight. Don't completely straighten your leg; this will put too much stress on your back.

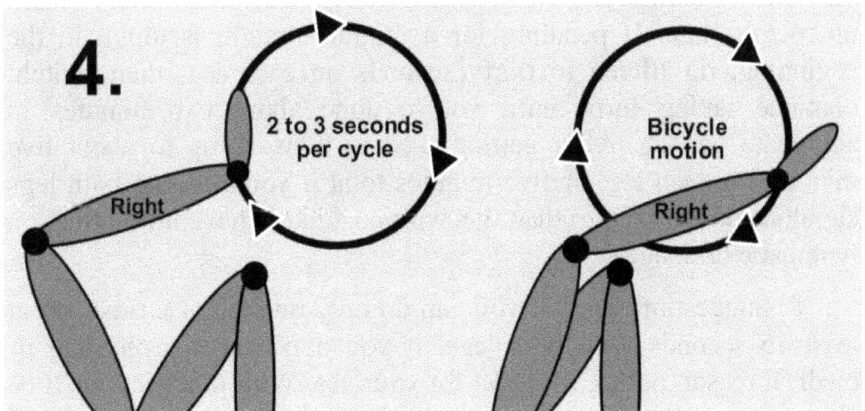

5. As you pedal, raise and lower your foot by flexing the calf muscles—point toe up, then point toe down. There is no necessity to establish any specific rhythm between your foot motions and how your move your legs, though one will generally develop on its own. This pumps the lymph from your foot and calf upward toward your thigh.

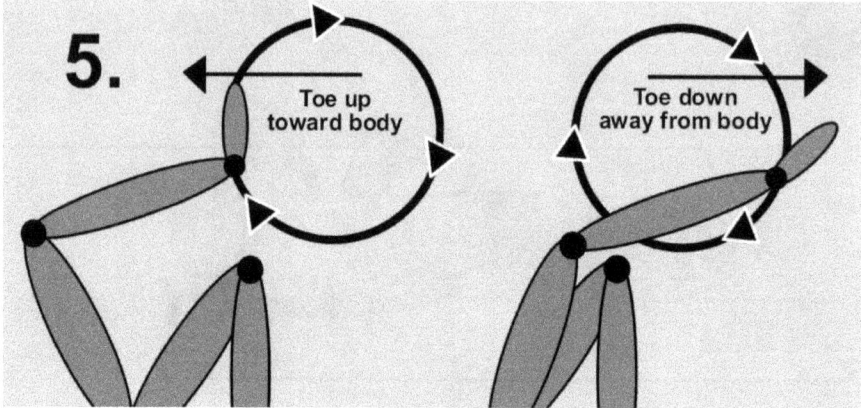

6. Don't move too quickly. Allow the fluids to travel; permit time for vessels to refill with lymph as it's pushed along. This is the most efficient way to do this exercise.

7. You should pedal one revolution every two to three seconds. This is a slow motion. Continue for about one minutes per leg, rest a moment if necessary, then do the other leg. You may have to work up to this time. If pedaling for a minute straight is tough in the beginning, do fifteen to thirty seconds on each leg, then switch; continue taking turns until you've done about two minutes in aggregate per leg. After getting used to it, work up to about five minutes on each leg, or five minutes total if you're doing both legs simultaneously. Longer than this will most likely have little effect on lymphatic drainage.

8. Suggestion: even if you can do only one leg at a time, try at least 15 seconds with both legs, if you don't have a physical or medical reason not to. It's great for your abs. With practice, you'll be able to work both legs simultaneously for the entire exercise and shorten the amount of time you invest in this procedure.

9. Do the exercise each morning and evening. If you don't have the time or patience to do both, then the evening is the better of the two. If you skip a day, there's no problem; this is as much art as science, but never just arbitrarily say, "I don't feel like it today." Each time you do that, you give your woman a free pass to say the same.

There are few men, other than those who get regular full-body exercise, who won't benefit from this exercise above-and-beyond the specific purpose of pumping life back into Harry. Do air cycling with your woman, she'll benefit as well.

TO REPEAT: Having gotten clearance from your physician, if at any time while doing this exercise, you feel faint, have trouble breathing, or experience back or any type of physical distress, or have chest pain, STOP. In the latter event, definitely call for assistance.

I'd like to add just a little more about the lymphatic system. This may not apply directly to our quest for a more reliable wanger, but it will help with some self-esteem issues if you tend to be overweight.

Water-weight, that bane of women during their period, is actually an accumulation of lymph in bodily tissues. The extra water that is retained is held partly in lymph. Water retention occurs when the body does not remove fluid from the tissues effectively. Fluid balance is controlled by hormones. A woman's hormones go through *the cycle* and many battle water-weight build up every month. But why men?

There are diseases that cause extreme water retention ranging from parasitic infection to cancer. Excessive build up or disfiguring swelling—not simply being "puffy"—should alert you to see your doctor immediately. However, in everyday situations where you may feel bloat throughout your body, simple water retention may be due to lack of exercise (the primary message of this chapter) plus poor diet.

Excessive salt intake is the most common reason for weight gain due to water retention in men. This will cause you to put on pounds and make you look inflated—dare I use the word "puffy" again? For most men, eliminating salt from the diet—or greatly reducing its intake—will cause rapid weight loss, including a reduction in waist size and visible improvement in one's appearance. This is the magic in many quick weight-loss programs: a drastic reduction in salt that guarantees a loss of pounds in days. But it's temporary if you go back to eating salty foods.

Reduction in salt intake should always be accompanied by an INCREASE in water consumption. Your kidneys will take care of the excess water as long as salt is not holding it in your body.

Lymph has to be pumped out of your tissues and the excess water has to move into your blood stream for it to be transported to your kidneys and peed away. That's why the exercise will assist anyone—ED or not—who goes through bouts of bloat.

Joke Time: This is an adaptation of a joke told by Mark Twain.
Patient: "If I give up red meat, smoking cigars, and drinking hard liquor, will I live longer?"
Doctor: "No, but it will seem that way."

I know that giving up, or even cutting down on salt means stripping your life of everything from nuts and pretzels—the staple of bar food—to almost everything else. But the connection between salt and water is not an on-off switch. One salty treat won't destroy your progress, but several days in a row will set you back.

I'm still convinced that the pressure of excess water has an effect on Harry's performance-biology by applying pressure to blood vessels and irritating nerves. Anything you can do to cut down on the number of pounds of salt you consume each month or week, will positively affect your overall health and that goes right to the little hanger.

There are other causes of water retention in men including, but not limited to, vitamin B1 (thiamine) insufficiency, certain other medications you may be taking including steroids and non-steroidal NSAIDs, and even sunburn and hot weather. If you have a rapid increase in water retention, see your doctor immediately. However, the number of men afflicted with non-salt related water retention is miniscule compared to the average Joe out there who lives on greasy, fried foods doused in salt.

We can summarize this entire section with the simple statement: You want to clear your blood, lymph, and tissues of toxins.

• You need to clean out your lymphatic system so that these poisons are moved into your blood where your liver and kidneys can deal with them appropriately.

• You need to keep the fluids moving, and that means you have to keep moving.

• You need to deal with certain dietary extravagances, and there will be ample discussion about that later on.

• And you need to do the air cycling exercise.

Chapter 13: The Spinal Connection

There is a muscle attached to the back of your spine that weaves its way to the front of your pelvis, and connects high on your thigh bone. It takes leverage from your spine, raising your legs as you walk. It's the primary muscle you use when you raise your legs to do the exercise described in the previous chapter and is often the muscle responsible for chronic lower back pain in people who spend their lives sitting or are otherwise inactive.

This is the Psoas muscle. Silent P, pronounced "So' az."

When you're seated, your psoas muscle is relaxed and rests at its shortest length. When the psoas is allowed to be relaxed most of the time—day after day—it actually shrinks in length. When you stand up straight, it no longer *comfortably* reaches between its two attachments, your spine and your thigh. Simply, it's being pulled tightly—too tightly.

Ever notice when you spend a lot of time on your feet your lower back starts to hurt? Holding your body erect keeps the psoas muscle stretched tightly. Shortened by routine sitting, it can't reach its physiologically correct length. It begins to ache.

So what does this have to do with Harry?

The psoas muscle connects the spine to the femur. It takes leverage off the spine to raise your legs when you walk or run, and especially when you climb stairs. However, your spine is not one big bone; it's a series of bones—vertebrae—that move relative to each other.

The spinal cord is that big channel of nerves that connects the brain to the rest of your body, including Harry. The spinal cord is housed within the protective walls of the vertebral bones that make up the spine. When your lover strokes you, the special nerves in Harry's head—nerve ending unlike any other in the body, thank you Lord—send the message, "She touched me!" along nerves from

Harry which are threaded through openings in the vertebrae. These nerves merge into the spinal cord and connect up to your brain.

Your brain interprets the "She touched me!" sensation as pleasurable, and stimulates the endocrine system to trigger nitric oxide production where it's needed for an erection. It also sends a command down the spinal cord. The nerves again exit the vertebrae through those small openings in the bones and travel to your penis. Harry snaps to attention.

Similarly, if you see your lover as she pulls the shower curtain back and steps dripping wet out of the tub to get a towel—she catches you watching, and smiles—a message will originate spontaneously in the brain which flies downs the spinal nerves that makes ol' one-eye look, too.

The part of this system that most concerns us right now is the communication between the sensory nerves in Harry, the spinal cord connection to the brain, and those nerves on the return route. The key is the clarity of the signal.

A Brief Review

• There are muscles in the arterial walls that control the flow of blood into the penis. These muscles are normally "on," closing the valve. These need a signal from the brain to be relaxed so that blood can be allowed to pump into Harry.

• There are muscles in the walls of the veins that control the flow of blood out of the penis. Normally "off," leaving the exit valve open, these need to be tightened to hold the blood in. Signals from the brain are essential for this, too.

• There are the "Thank you, Lord" nerve endings in the head of the penis which keep that blessed sensation going as long as possible until they ultimately get the "I can't hold back anymore" signal from the brain to let-'er-rip.

• Then there are the nerves to the stomach that tell the brain, "Boy, I could go for some pizza and a beer 'bout now."

Each of these functions is controlled by the brain and must have an open and uninterrupted signal from the right subinsular region including the left caudate, claustrum, and putamen, bilateral cingulate gyrus, right middle occipital/middle temporal gyri, and right sensorimotor and premotor regions of the brain.

Got all that?

Basically, there's a lot of stuff going on to get Harry happy. Uninterrupted and unhampered signals to and from your brain are necessary. You can have the best HDTV in the world, but if you're using a composite instead of HDMI connection, you're not going to get a clean signal from your digital box.

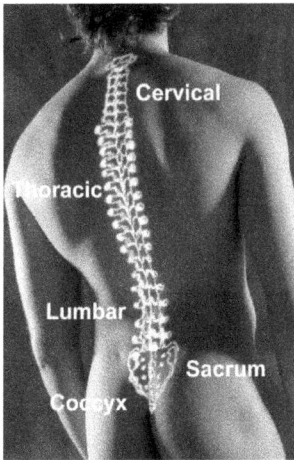

Irritated nerves react by becoming inflamed. The signals they send become fuzzy images, and that's about as far as I'm going to go with this analogy. It would be so much easier to explain if we still used antennas for televisions.

The nerves that lead to Harry come down the spinal cord and exit the spine in the area called the sacrum. The sacrum is actually five bones that are naturally fused into one. It is located just above the coccyx, or the "tail bone," at the very bottom of the spine.

The spinal cord itself—the major nerve bundle—ends at the bottom of the lumbar region of the spine which is just above the sacrum. The nerves travel down the spine into the lower lumbar vertebrae and then leave the spinal cord and continue into the sacrum. There, they exit through holes in the sacrum and begin their journey through soft tissue to Harry.

Remember the psoas? It latches onto the spine in the lumbar region. When it's too tight, it contorts the spine which can create pressure on these nerves. The psoas doesn't have to be in full-blown spasm; you don't have to be bent over in debilitating pain for it to do its dirty work. Just a moderate contraction of the psoas causes curvature, stresses the spinal column, and creates a misalignment—a subluxation—of the vertebrae.

Like an electrical wire exiting a conduit, if the conduit is moved after the wire is drawn, its edge can be abrasive on the wire. The nerves that normally exit the spine cleanly and without undue contact with the bone can become irritated when rubbed against the vertebrae due to the distortion caused by psoas contraction. The nerve is a living cell. It continues to function, but because of the irritation, it may not communicate information up or down the spinal cord as well as it should. The pressure on the nerve may only cause a mild irritation that you may not notice with any discernible sensation... until, well... you call upon Harry.

2010. I had a comfortable chair at my desk, and like most days, I was stationary for hours. One afternoon, after pounding on my computer non-stop until mid-afternoon, I finished a project, saved the file, rolled my chair back, and without second thought, attempted to stand. Halfway up, my back locked. I mean LOCKED!

I carefully lowered back down; the pain was so great I couldn't breathe. When the agony subsided, I carefully rose, measuring each inch as a conquest. I hobbled to my car and headed to the chiropractor. After an examination, he gave me over to the massage therapist. The manipulation was painful. She moved me and pressed me and bent me and elbowed me. By the end of the hour, I was feeling a little better, but still a far way from being fixed.

The diagnosis: spasm of the psoas. The muscle had locked up so fiercely that it compressed my lumbar vertebrae against my sacrum causing excruciating pain.

I visited his office I visited his office daily, and felt much better after the fourth day. He showed me the Psoas stretch (discussed next) which, candidly, I couldn't do for a week until I was able to comfortably lower myself to one knee.

This all happened in the same time frame as my ED; I was particularly attentive to my sexual sensations, or lack thereof, as a completely separate matter from my back issues. Harry started to rejoin my team as I worked with my chiropractor and massage therapist to relive my psoas issues.

With my background in biology and physiology, I began contemplating why, as my chronic pain went away, my member came back to life. At first I thought it was just a pain thing; the pain in my back referring down to Harry—it's hard to get hard when you're hurting. With some further research, I put the spine-nerve-pecker connection together and added it to my hypotheses.

Stretching Your Psoas

If my hypothesis is correct, stretching the psoas muscle will eliminate yet another factor contributing to your erectile dysfunction. If my hypothesis is wrong, you'll still get rid of a lot of annoying back pain, so either way, you should stretch your psoas muscle.

One way to begin is to get a therapeutic massage, for which I am a strong proponent. A good therapist, when asked, will work the psoas, relaxing and elongating it to its optimum length. She will also help stimulate movement of lymph and removal of toxins (lactic acid and others) from your muscles furthering the previous chapter's objectives.

Whether or not you get a massage, this is a stretching exercise you can do at home or work to quickly remediate this muscle.

The Psoas Stretch is a common exercise recommended by many massage and physical therapists, and chiropractors. There are a number of versions. All are acceptable, and whichever one you choose, it will be very helpful for both men and women. You can find videos of the various stretches available on the Internet: Google "Psoas Stretch" and you'll come up with several high-ranking hits for YouTube files that clearly demonstrate the procedure.

I'm going to describe the version that works for me.

As always, you must not have any issues which will be aggravated by the exercise. Be wary of any preexisting conditions with your knees, hips, or back. Check with your doctor, orthopedist, or chiropractor. Again, use common sense.

The Psoas Stretch

1. Get down on your left knee with your right foot flat on the floor—the basic "Will you marry me?" position. Try not to hyperventilate, this is only pretend.

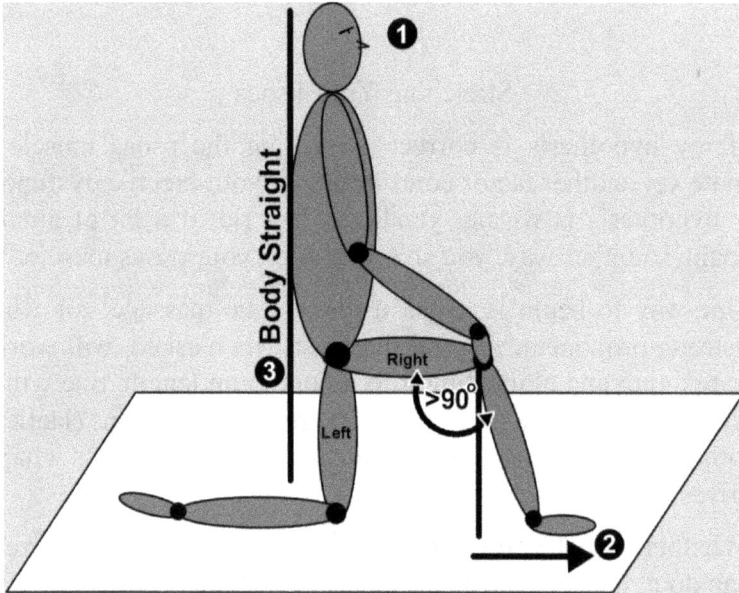

2. Move your right foot, the one on the floor, forward about 8 inches without moving or changing the angle of your left leg. The angle of your right leg—calf to thigh—should be greater than a right angle, that is, more than 90 degrees.

3. Your back should be straight.

4. Pull yourself forward using your right leg: close your right leg until the right calf is 90 degrees or less relative to your right thigh. Your left knee should not have moved on the floor. You should feel tension in the front of your left thigh muscle—the quadriceps.

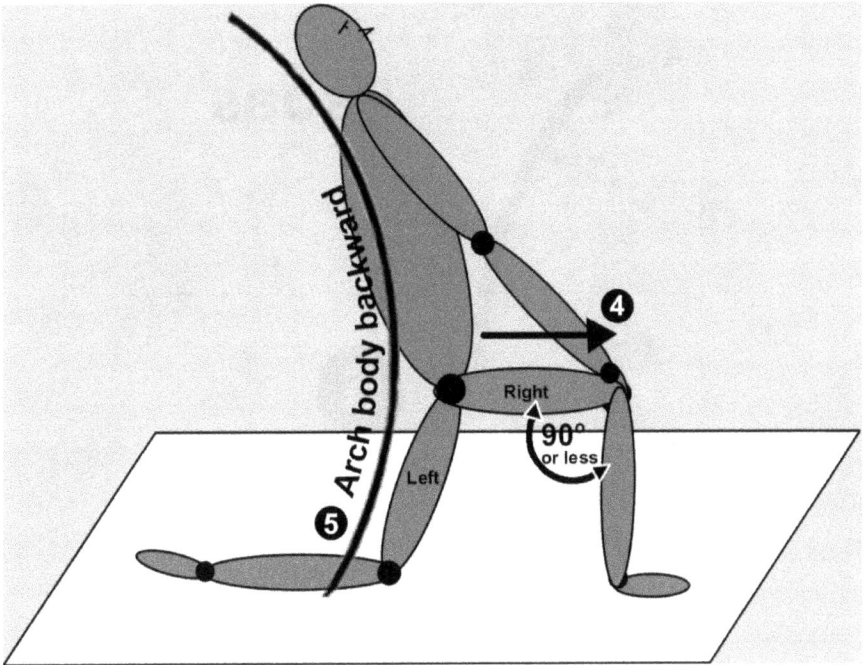

5. At the same time, arch yourself backwards as far as you can. Try to look straight up at the ceiling without bending your head very far back. Do the best you can. Your tight psoas will be fighting you and you may not be able to go back very far when you first try the exercise. Over time, you'll do better.

6. The idea is to bend your thigh back relative to your spine as far as you can thereby stretching the psoas muscle that connects the two. The psoas has to round the bend at your pelvis and is stretched taught. Don't overdue to start. Like everything else, this takes time.

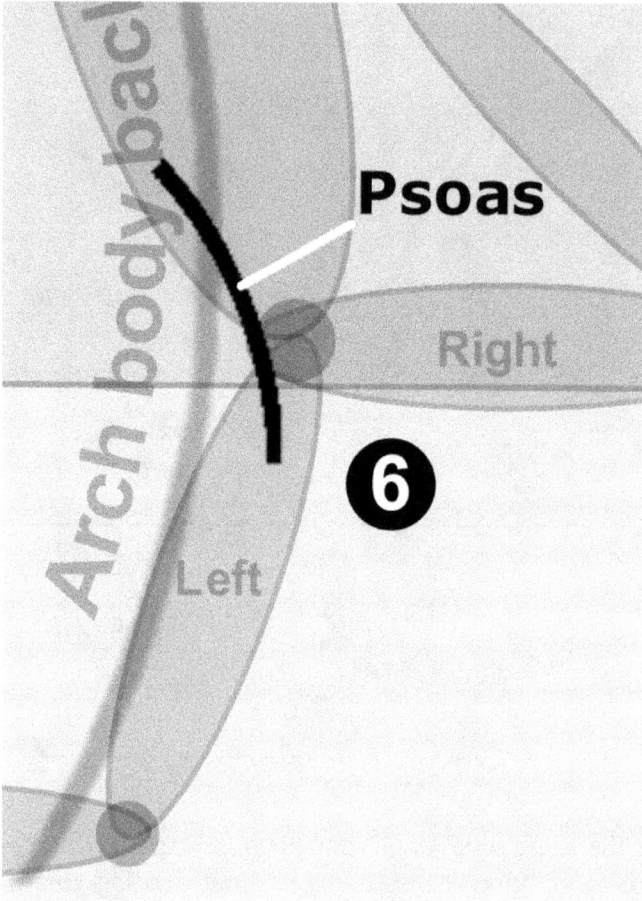

7. It is okay to push with your arms or have a friend pull you backward—gently—at the shoulders. While you should feel tension in your muscles, it should not be painful. And don't be disheartened if you can't stretch back very far when you first start—that's just means you really need it.

8. Hold for a full 20 seconds. Don't cheat or you'll only be cheating yourself.

9. Relax for a few seconds, change legs and repeat with your right knee on the floor.

10. Repeat doing 20 seconds, 3 times on each knee. *Do not aggregate*, that is, do not do 60 seconds on each knee. You must alternate for periods not to exceed about 20 seconds.

11. It is best to do this exercise, as with most, several hours after you've gotten out of bed. For most people that's 10:00AM or later.

12. Stretch twice or three times a day as you can. Do it every day. Try it right now as you're reading this.

13. Do this as a stretch before the air pedaling exercise described in the previous chapter. It's a very effective pre-sex stretch as well—for both of you.

14. Even when things are going well, and Harry is working consistently and effectively, and you have no back pain, it is wise to stretch at least once each day just to stay in shape.

15. The entire exercise, including the switch from one knee to the other, only steals about 2-1/2 minutes of your time!

To reconstitute the psoas muscle to its natural length, perform the psoas stretch with regularity. Your back will feel better. This will motivate you to do other physical activities and improve the overall quality of your life. I'm not exaggerating. Remove even a few of the body pains that you "just live with," and you will elevate your mood and life.

Air cycling and the psoas stretch: I spend ten minutes every day doing things that may keep Harry happy for years to come.

Chapter 14: The Mind is a Terrible Thing

We're going to deal with some psychological issues, inasmuch as even a slight reduction in physical ability due to poor lifestyle is so very amplified by what goes on in that vast unknown region of the Male Psyche.

That specific stress—Performance Anxiety—associated with transitory impotence is the brunt of jokes and television sitcoms. The embarrassment of "It happens to every guy…" is not made easier by "…once in a while," when you're in the middle of that while.

I have no easy fix. Sometimes a drink or two works to take the edge off. But I admit freely, that if Charlize Theron—a particular heart-throb of mine—showed up at my door, took me by my hand and led me to the bedroom... I just don't know what would happen. From premature ejaculation—while she was still ringing the doorbell—to total erectile failure, the scenario is unpredictable. But maybe, just maybe, if I'm in good enough physical shape endowing me with full confidence, I could initiate some great lovemaking and carry it through to both our satisfaction.

I know that if I'm having ED issues before she shows up at my door, the added stress will leave me stranded like a cracked engine block.

I recently had a conversation with a longtime friend who questioned his own ability to perform. He's in the throes of a bloody divorce at the inevitable conclusion of a marriage that has been without intimacy for a long time. He doesn't know if he has a problem, he hasn't had the chance to try in quite a while. But, as part of discussing how much he'd like to find a woman once the legalities of his marriage are concluded, he voiced his concern over whether he'd have difficulties when he has his opportunity to get in the saddle.

All by itself, I informed him, asking the question is the first step to ensuring that there *will* be a problem. He's got to get it out of his mind.

Anxiety Equals Stress, and Stress Kills.

Stress raises blood pressure—the systolic (lower number) which is the real killer. Systolic, your resting pressure in between heart beats, is also raised when blood vessels are hardened and they don't flex or dilate as well as they must.

Where have we run into blood vessel dilation before? Nitric oxide. Stress releases molecules into your general circulation that destroys nitric oxide. No **NO**, No go.

Temporary stress can do the same, subjecting us to that "once in a while" we guys dread. But a continual flood of stress can so destroy the nitric oxide producing mechanism of the body that it could take months to heal.

Don't let yourself get to that state by allowing stress, plus all the chemicals, acids, and irritants attack your blood vessels. Stress alone is a formidable foe in the fight for potency. Remove the chemicals and it gets less destructive, and while cleansing one's body of chemicals can takes weeks or months, stress can be wiped away with just a change of attitude.

Granted, that's way easier said than done.

E. D.—Erectile Dystopia

When you perceive yourself to be caught in a miserable day-to-day routine, it can be summed up in just two words, "Life sucks," and that can go straight to your dick.

When all seems to fail around you, your marriage, your job, your relationship with your kids, plus you're a Cubs fan, at least there's one thing left; you still have that one chance in a million that you might somewhere, somehow, in some place at some time... well... you might get laid.

Ironically, just at that time, Harry leaves the building. Why? Perhaps:

- You're in a *bad/failing/failed* marriage. Choose one, and;

- You have to deal with a *bastard boss/son-of-a bitch coworkers/asshole clients.* Choose all that apply, and;
- Your kids are *irresponsible/disrespectful/demanding.* Select all, and;
- Your investments are in the toilet.

What did you expect?

I described how physical sensation is detected by those very wonderful nerves that cover the head of the penis. A chemical-electrical image of those sensations is transmitted through nerves to the spinal cord and then up to the brain that quickly interprets them. The brain then initiates a series of signals down the nerves which, if the machinery is working properly, initiates and sustains an erection.

For all the unwanted, inappropriate and mostly just badly-timed hard-ons we had throughout our teens and twenties, we men find ourselves stymied by just the opposite later in our years. Just as chemical toxins can accumulate in our blood, toxic thoughts can aggregate in our minds. These poisonous psychic fancies deaden Harry as quickly as a shot of Novocain.

Of course there are the big notions. In a marriage, you may question, *Does she even care anymore,* or *Is she just waiting for me to finish?* In a new relationship you may wonder, *Am I as big as her last lover?* And then there are other issues, *Whoa, was he talking about a shot of Novocain in my dick?*

During-sex thoughts can quickly shut Harry down. More insidious are the myriad little worries about money, job, spousal approval of one's adequacy as a parent, money, the kids, the toilet won't flush, money, the gutters of the house need cleaning, did I mention money? These wear on a man and make sexual performance difficult. It is reasonable to say that many of you reading this book wish you had the balls to run away to Tahiti, find a wonderful young, bare-breasted beauty and just pick coconuts and fuck daily until you die. That, by the way, would be Tuesday; Tahitian men don't like paunchy guys from Newark showing up to pork their women.

When a woman is distracted by the pressures and obligations of her life, she may be prone to a loss of libido from her state of mind. Women say, "Not tonight." She is difficult to arouse and often will refuse to try. Some experience *frigidity,* including an inability to self-lubricate. However, when something that she feels is romantic strikes—you say or do the right thing at the right time—she could snap back into action and be fully engaged in the moment.

Likewise, a man's psyche, in the absence of any of the aforementioned chemical assaults on the body, can leave him dysfunctional. It can occur to varying degrees and can inhibit some or all attempts at play. It will happen at the worst possible time. You will discover it after a long absence of sexual intimacy. You get into bed and it's just not there.

Want to test whether you've got a strong psychological component to your ED? Next time you masturbate—yes, your birthday is coming soon—take note of how many times your mind wanders to the mundane—the house, the bills, your job. You practically have to fight your way back to your happy place to finish the task at hand.

Thank you, Joseph Heller. *Catch 22* is illustrated no better place than in the bedroom. You're under stress and can't get it up, but if you could just get it up you could release some of the stress.

It's all cumulative.

There have been some dramatic advances in neurophysiology and biochemistry in the past several decades. Researchers tell us that the chemicals responsible for our moods and feelings are not just present in our brains, but in every cell of our bodies.

Of course, your organs don't smile, laugh, or cry. They express their mood by the way they perform. A person who's having a stressful, anxious day, may suffer indigestion or a headache. A body drowning from the inside in molecules of unhappiness, anxiety, and depression day after week after month, is going to spiral downward. There's an impact on the health of every organ. Inflammation spreads. The immune system is weakened, opening up the body to all manner of disease, dysfunction, and cancer. Most heart attacks happen on Monday mornings—such is the power of the emotion of dread.

While ED should be the least of your health worries, it's the most apparent and goes to the top of the list. Sex is often what makes us feel most like men—at least for a while—and sex releases immune boosting emotion molecules which heal. A guy who is well-laid generally feels better for much of the day.

As a sufferer of ED, you must make yourself feel better about yourself and your life's situation. Easier said than done? Perhaps it is, but not so difficult to do, if you'd just give it a try.

If you're coming off a long hiatus, or you're newly divorced, or perhaps trying to reconnect with your significant other, it's the *not knowing if you'll perform* that causes anxiety. Here's where taking a pill has validity, at least it did for me.

As described much earlier, I knew I had a problem. I did my research. Having formulated my hypothesis, I followed the practices I've laid out in this book. I was pretty sure, based on the way I felt that I was ready to get back into action. Still, I did not know for sure, so I got a prescription. When a lady extended an invitation to me, I took the pill, and performed admirably. My partner never knew.

I could have taken a freaking sugar pill, but my perception that "I was covered" was all I needed and the anxiety was gone. I started with a full dose for the first time, then I cut to half before going sober and straight.

But what if your stress is real? What if it is a product of concrete, situational challenges, not some imaginary anxiety issues?

A common example: you're in a relationship from which you cannot easily extricate yourself—married with children and a prenup—or you simply choose not to leave because you feel the marriage can be salvaged. You've got to work to reduce or eliminate the marital discord first. Begin immediately. Time does not *heal all* once a relationship is solidly on the rocks.

When you turn your relationship around, then you should feel better about yourself and Harry may very well cooperate spontaneously.

I'm not a marriage counselor and profess no special training or knowledge regarding the resolution of well entrenched marital trials and tribulations, but I do live in the real world. I pose a scenario in which you have a conversation with your wife or partner. At the very least, the answer to the final question can be critical in determining your life's path.

"Wife [replace with a formal or cutesy name as applicable], I'd like to get into shape. I want to feel better about myself and I'm hoping you'll help. If I really gave it a try, will you help me?"

"Yeah, right," she says. *You're losing her attention, so don't hesitate; charge right in.*

"Yes I am! I'm too young to give up sex for the rest of my life. I want to get into shape sufficient to have sex comfortably, and you're the one I want to have sex with." *Pause and wait for her response. Don't oversell it. Just wait.*

She looks at you like you're crazy, but you've got her attention—or disdain.

"I'm going to do this. I know the last time we tried it just didn't work well. It's because I'm way out of shape. I want to get healthy enough that it'll come back and when it does I want to make love to you. Just tell me. Is there any circumstance where you would ever want to make love to me again?"

I know one guy who got the answer, "No." He's completed a no-fault divorce and he and his ex-wife are both happier living separately. They both have new partners, too.

I don't know the state of your relationship, whether the feeling she had for you—or the two of you for each other—still exists or not. If it doesn't, consider divorce, have an affair, or resign yourself to life-long abstinence, or self-gratification.

I am sure there are certain demographics within American society that could never have this conversation; the discussion of wanting sex for the intrinsic pleasure of it outside of the intention to procreate, simply could never happen. I am also pretty sure that the people in those niches of our society are not reading this book.

If she says "No," then you know your options.

However, if there's any spark of possibility, she has to give you some credit for raising the question. It has to make her think. And you've just taken the first step toward getting Harry back on the team. Hell, you've just taken the first step to getting back your team.

But if she remembers the good times and gives you a shot it, it may be your last. Ya gotta follow through. Don't fuck it up!

Performance Anxiety

It's clichéd that a new relationship can be impacted by just worrying about whether you can *do it* or not. But PA can come into play when trying to renew sexual intimacy within an existing relationship as well. And PA gangs up with all the other psychological, physical, chemical, and nutritional stressors to leave you limp.

If you're otherwise in great shape and enjoy a healthy diet, psychological stress can be the single reason for ED; don't ignore that possibility. Professional counseling to address your psyche and reinforce your self-confidence should not be overlooked whether you're trying to renew a romance with your long-term lover, or you have difficulties with new ones.

The mind and body are more interactive than most traditional medical practitioners understand. Eating well, eliminating toxic chemicals, increasing vegetables, decreasing meat protein and fat, and getting some modicum of exercise will affect your state of mind, giving you mental, physical, and penile vitality.

Earl Nightingale, in his monumental work, *Lead the Field*, presents an analysis of worry. I strongly recommend this recorded program for you and your children, whether teens or adults. To paraphrase, he demonstrates that only eight percent of things that people worry about are worth worrying about with ninety-two percent being a complete waste of energy and angst. They include worries about which you have no control, and worries about things that never subsequently happen.

With just a few percentage points of legitimate worries, if you don't have the motivation to do what needs to be done to avoid or prepare for the fated outcome, then—I have to wonder—why worry about them either?

Have you ever shown up at work on a dark, rainy day to find that everyone looks and feels *down?* Their energy levels are low and they look like they just don't feel well. Someone might say, "It must be the weather." They'd be right. Some aspect of the increased humidity, drop in barometric pressure, reduction in outdoor light affects the way we feel, but it doesn't have to.

Some do not experience this short-lived depression at all, and if you make note of who they are, you'll find they're the people who are generally in better spirits all the time; they are working from a higher platform.

You can even get an indication of someone's mind-set by listening to the words they use. Such is the condition that it has been captured in cliché as a common human experience; those "under the weather" will call the day, gloomy or dismal. Those who have a more positive outlook tend to agree with poet and songwriter Rod McKuen who once said about a rainy afternoon, "It's a great day to get into bed with a good book... or somebody who's read one."

If something as simple as the weather with which we deal every day affects us, how can you not expect to have the more aggressive demands of life fail to take their toll? All the external influences to which we are subjected—political vitriol, pressures from the pulpit, the demands of Madison Avenue—these all accumulate in your mind like sewage in a septic tank. You have to take the initiative to pump it out, or it's going to cost you a bundle.

In terms of your health, stress pounds the hell out of your immune system and will make you susceptible to disease and dysfunction, in addition to going straight to Harry.

Some Tips on Releasing the Pressures of Stress

Remember W. C. Fields' joke, "I feel sorry for anyone who doesn't drink. When they get up in the morning, that's as good as they're going to feel all day." I said that you shouldn't give up drinking, unless, of course, you find it very easy to do so.

Getting together with family and friends to eat and drink is a staple of most cultures. It's as important to health as the good food and clean water you drink. Camaraderie, laughter, and good times save lives. People who don't find the time to enjoy life will suffer, not only immediately, but also later on.

Only wholesome, loving sex is better for health. An orgasm stimulates your endocrine system to release hormones throughout your body that promote mental and physical health and create a feeling of well-being that extends well beyond the act itself. And love will do for an orgasm what Bose speakers does for an iPod.

Touch & Laughter

The simple act of touching begins to fine-tune your body for sex, so don't hurry through your love making desperate for the endorphin rush. Caress and care; every moment in which you touch each other adds some amount of time to your lives, and you don't have to wait until you're in bed.

Hold hands, sit side-by-side on the couch, massage each other's feet. It all counts toward extending your time here, and it feels so good while you're doing it. It overcomes psychological obstacles to a substantial erection, and dilates the blood vessels—the same thing many ED pills do—and puts your metabolism in harmony. Touch and affection are good for Harry.

So much has been written about laughter that it may be unnecessary to reiterate, but laughter promotes health. If you're sick it will heal you. If you have systemic inflammation, it can reduce the effects of the irritation throughout your body—though not all by itself.

As a health therapy, watching funny movies or going to comedy clubs is a great start. But there's much more. You have to allow yourself to laugh.

When one is in a bad mood, nothing seems funny. Everyone around will be in fits of hysterical laughter and that one person will have exiled him or herself from the party. If you are one of those people who is perennially in a bad mood—and you have a thousand bullshit excuses as to why you must be—then you have to lighten your heart so that you find more things funny. That's not a girly thing to do. It's a human thing.

- Improve your diet by following as many of the preceding advice points as you possibly can. Bad mood is often a result of bad diet. General body pain or malaise is a sign of poor nutrition and originates in the digestive tract.
- You may feel like shit because you're literally full of shit. Eat some greens, have some fruit, dump regularly.
- Because you feel bad, you just can't bring yourself to exercise. You don't exercise, so you feel even more like crap. It's yet another incarnation of Catch-22.

Put the cycle in reverse. Do something. Get off your ass. Get some exercise. You'll feel better, and feeling better will motivate you to do more. You are in control!

Meditation versus Contemplation

Those of you who can effectively meditate should continue to do so—though you don't need my permission. Nothing I say here is meant to denigrate the art and practice of meditation or imply that it is not a valid stress-relieving, spirit-enlightening modality.

A quick explanation of meditation for the Western practitioner: One sits in a quiet, comfortable place. Eyes are closed and the mind is emptied. Should a thought come into one's mind, like a leaf floating in a stream, one is to let it continue on its journey and pass out of one's mental view. With some—considerable—practice, one should be able to clear one's mind of all the mundane thoughts of one's life and achieve a state of perfect, restful tranquility.

I prefer contemplation. I relax out on the deck of my small suburban home with a glass of scotch in one hand, a small, quality cigar in the other, and I stare out at the trees watching the squirrels and birds play and forage for food. Occasionally a humming bird comes by or a chipmunk scurries past my feet.

I sit and think. If I have a specific problem that's weighing on my mind, I mull over all things I know about it, sip some whisky, take a puff on the stogie, and try to figure out what I can do to resolve the issue. Other thoughts may come into my mind. Some I dismiss and others I deal with right then and there. I usually have a pad and pencil available should I have an idea that I wish to preserve in its native form.

Let me give you an example of a time when one stressful and disturbing problem needed to be addressed without any delay: My dick didn't work.

Much of the first work—the hypothesis and the strategy, and my *AHA!* moment described earlier—was a result of numerous evenings staring at the trees and thinking.

The object of contemplation is to think, to initiate new thoughts from within, to create mental links between those facts, presumptions, and speculations that are already known, and in doing so arrive at something new.

Often, I'd make notes on what I wished to Google when I went back to my computer; my personal practice was NOT to have my electronics with me so as not to be distracted.

As a result of my contemplations, I formalized a plan, took action, further refined the process, and then put the lead back in my pencil—both literally and euphemistically. You're reading my report.

All by itself, the process of working toward a solution of a problem reduces the internal stress cascade that has impact on your life and that of Harry. Certainly, when you find a solution, or even just devise a plan of action to alleviate the situation, you feel much better.

I've worked through numerous problems with varying levels of success. Sometimes, the very clever thoughts at which I arrived by working on some problem through contemplation don't lead to a useful solution. However, even on those occasions, I did have a restful, stress-relieving hour or so out on my deck with the birds and the squirrels and my brown liquor and my cigar. Gotta love it.

Author's note: The next sections regarding your adrenal glands, cortisol, hormones, and your liver cross the boundary between psychological issues—the primary topic of this chapter—and physical/metabolic assaults on the body. There is no way to legitimately separate one's mental state from hormone production, especially in the arena of male sexual health, so these subjects are necessarily interlaced.

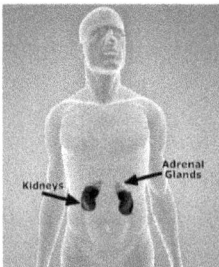

Adrenal Glands and Adrenal Health

The adrenal glands are two small walnut-sized organs that sit on top of your kidneys. Even the non-biologists among you probably recognize the adrenal glands as the producers of adrenalin.

Adrenalin is the "fight or flight" hormone that gets your heart pumping and muscles tensed. Evolutionarily, it allowed our ancestors to quickly respond to a critical situation by either fighting off a threat, or fleeing from the danger. Today it produces road-rage.

In addition to adrenalin, these glands also produce other hormones including cortisol, a small amount of testosterone, and building blocks for other hormones. According to Dr. James Wilson who made popular the term "Adrenal Fatigue," the adrenal glands, "...modulate the functioning of every tissue, organ and [other] glands in your body to maintain homeostasis during stress *and keep you alive.*" *Emphasis* by author.

As stated earlier, every cell in our bodies has the ability to express itself by creating and secreting mood molecules into our systems. They also have the ability to receive instruction from circulating hormones and then respond to those instructions. That's exactly what hormones are for.

When you watch the nightly news and see the pathetic stupidity of the irrelevant and malevolent rants of a politician, your psyche stimulates your adrenal glands to produce adrenalin. The more you watch, the more it produces. Are you a politics junkie? Then, you've been dosed with unnecessary and damaging stress that has been tearing you apart for years (decades?). That holds true regardless of which side of the aisle your team sits. It applies, more recently, even if you're Canadian.

While you're staring at the tube with your adrenalin levels at high tide, your blood pressure rises. Every cell in your body is on alert. Your brain and body don't really know what to expect. Is there a saber-toothed tiger out there?

Fighting or flighting—physical activity—burns off the adrenaline, the associated neurotransmitters, and any number of naturally produced psychotropic compounds.

Without a physical reaction to adrenaline,
your body stews in a tension marinade.

This effect on every cell in your body pounds away at your libido, metabolically. The negative impact on your body of just a few minutes of talking heads during your news program continues long after the local weather has come and gone from the screen.

So you no longer have to wonder why Harry slumbers off before your favorite late night comedian walks onto the stage to yet again remind you—albeit humorously—of all the ills of the day via a monologue.

It beats the hell out of Harry both physiologically and psychologically.

Cortisol and Stress

Some stress is good-stress; psychologists call that *eustress*—"eu" from the Greek for "well" or "good." The opposite is *distress*—no explanation needed.

Distress, in Western society, is the product of the nonsense to which we subject ourselves for no reason whatsoever, except for those things you rationalize and make up excuses and alibis to justify. It's all shit. It's the 92% of worry that has no basis.

Watch much late night television? Surf the web? You've seen the infomercials and banner-ads for pills and supplements that will bring down your cortisol level to get rid of your belly fat. Cortisol is an important steroidal hormone that regulates essential processes within the body. We need it. It is produced by the body and is not something that we ingest with our food, and it is created by the adrenal glands in response to stress. Cortisol is needed for fat metabolism. It moves fat and energy stores to the place in the body where it's needed when it's needed, such as moving fat to large muscles during exercise so it can be burned up—that's the good stress.

Distress causes excess cortisol production. Cortisol fucks up. It starts moving fat to the visceral areas of your body, around your stomach and intestines. This internal accumulation of fat is much harder to access and takes a lot more work to lose. We've all seen the guy whose belt buckles point straight down as he continues to wear size 36 pants around a size 46 belly.

Hence, the term "belly fat." This term is bandied about by those who seek to entice you to buy their anti-cortisol pills.

You may ask, "What is the relevance of this to our discussion of psychological factors in ED?" Answer: Stress deadens Harry.

I rarely watch the news. The result is that I'm finding it much easier to lose weight. I've done everything, in fact, that is possible to reduce the stress in my life and I'm finally starting to improve my appearance and health—something I failed to be able to do on several previous attempts in the absence of stress modulation.

Cortisol doesn't make fat; it repositions it to areas of your body that won't burn off easily. Take heed—both men and women—it's the accumulation of internal fat that kills you. It's not the double or triple chin, or the cellulite on your legs, or your fat ass and thighs. It's the fat that surrounds and strangles your heart and other internal organs that's deadly.

And men, it also causes pressure on sensitive areas of your erectile machinery and can contribute to erectile dysfunction.

Remember erectile dysfunction? I haven't mentioned it in a few pages, but that's where we're heading with this discussion of the adrenal glands. Cortisol is first. Adrenal burn-out is second.

If you're under stress—real or imaginary—week after week, after year, it tires your adrenal glands, and it disrupts your entire endocrine system—your hormone balance—and both men and woman can experience the effect of loss of libido and sexual function.

For me, in addition to cleaning up my eating habits, minimizing stress was essential to help get the other aspects of my healthy lifestyle in gear. Reducing stress could not have done the job by itself, but as a factor in my recovery, it was significant.

Weight Loss

Reducing stress will reduce the rapidity with which you are gaining weight. As described, stress screws up cortisol production and puts the most deadly kind of weight on. The changes in diet described so far are not about slimming down, although with the modifications to your eating with the addition of a regular exercise regimen you will take off a few pounds and perhaps a few inches over time. That, plus dealing with stress will make you feel better.

Improvements in body strength and stamina will energize you. You will do more things in general and more of them with your woman. You relationship will improve. She might consider getting out there and walking with you, on the outside chance that she may need a bit of firming-up, too. If you're eating better, she will as well, along with the kids, if they're still at home.

Your life will still be plagued with money issues, job issues, kid issues, and with regularity, some mindless conflict that hits you from left field. But working from a higher platform, these will all be mitigated; they will be surmountable, which will leave you in a position to be "Sir Mountable."

A Segue to Testosterone

We all know that testosterone is the hormone that makes men, men. In the womb, we all start out as females. The production of testosterone in fetuses destined to become males changes the growing body to produce male reproductive organs and body features instead of those characteristic of females.

The testes produce most of the testosterone. The adrenal glands produce a little, but more importantly, they produce androgens, building blocks of other hormones including those necessary for testosterone. Interestingly, your balls drink cholesterol to make testosterone. Unfortunately, the presence of more cholesterol in your blood does not increase the amount of testosterone produced by the guys.

Adrenal health is essential to male health and performance for other reasons. The adrenals are just one of a trio of glands of the endocrine system that regulate most of what goes on in your body. The hypothalamus and pituitary are the others. The health—or lack thereof—of the adrenals, impacts these other glands.

The hypothalamus produces a hormone that stimulates the pituitary to produce other hormones that cause the testes to start converting cholesterol to testosterone. When testosterone is produced it's normally attached to a carrier molecule produced by the liver, which keeps it from doing anything—your body needs unattached testosterone to circulate in the blood and make everything work, so the amount of carrier molecule that's available regulates how much testosterone you have wandering around doing testosterone things.

It's all so freaking complicated! Everything is connected to everything else!

> *Excess adrenal load due to distress, in concert with overworking your liver by poor dietary habits, affects the ability of your body to produce the most important chemical activator of your sex drive and erection-producing mechanism.*

> *plus*

> *Erectile dysfunction, as a stressor in and of itself, creates more ED biochemically, further augmented by the psychological factors discussed earlier.*

Simply, stress, whether it's over money, the kids, or your job will take its toll on your dick. Add to that the completely irrelevant nonsense on the news, and the outrage over the color the neighbor painted his house, and the asshole that just couldn't drive at the speed limit and keep up with traffic... the perception of all this bathes our minds and bodies in the biochemical equivalent of stress. No wonder there are more than thirty million men in the United States who suffer some degree of erectile dysfunction.

Just to backpedal for a moment—there is some good stress. The events that upset, *and motivate us,* don't cause the kind of internal disruptions that I'm describing. Rationally taking action—addressing that which we perceive as stressful—neutralizes the negative effects on our bodies. *It's the things that upset us over which we feel we have no control* that weaken Harry and can kill us.

It's the long term stress—months, years, decades—that tears up Harry. That's why ED is predominately, though not exclusively, an affliction of those over fifty. It takes that long. Fortunately, it can be reversed and the bulk of this book describes what you have to do to chart a new course. Exercise is key. It is the best mechanism to burn off the worry and stress that attacks your ability to produce testosterone.

Getting your lungs and heart going with even so much as a healthy walk—one brisk enough to increase your heart rate and respiration—just a few times a week can begin to help bring Harry back from the dead.

Physical exertion, as when playing sports or having sex actually increases the production of testosterone.

More: Estrogen suppresses the production of testosterone. The male body produces a little bit of estrogen, too, though not enough to understand *mauve.* The hormones used on meat and poultry—whose only purpose is to enhance corporate profit—include estrogen. That estrogen is still present in the meat when you eat it. It can contribute to "Low T," a newly coined term by a pharmaceutical company that now provides—surprise, surprise—a drug to combat this newly invented disease.

Unfortunately, alcohol reduces testosterone levels, too. Specifically, beer contains plant versions of estrogens that are pharmacologically active in humans and can reduce testosterone production in men.

PART III: General Health Issues & Things that Affect Harry

Chapter 15: V.O.D. — Vital Organ Dysfunction

Adrenal Glands II

We've discussed your adrenal glands, their function in erectile health, relationship to other glands of your endocrine—hormone—system, and how psychological stress can reduce their effectiveness.

These glands are responsible for maintaining your life, not just your sex life. It's not just stress that fatigues these organs. The entire spectrum of artificial foods, chemicals, dyes, and stimulants also beat them up. But there's one big gun that we aim at our adrenals just to start our day… Caffeine … that elevates adrenal function. The *jittery* you feel on a high-volume coffee day is not directly from the caffeine, it's the adrenalin produced by your adrenal glands as a reaction to the caffeine. That's what is stimulated by the stimulant.

Too much coffee stresses your adrenals, causes weight gain, and hampers your ability to deal with minor events in your life, all of which impact Harry. So how much is okay? A cup or two early in the day is best. Stop drinking coffee after about three PM. If you need more, or enjoy a cup after dinner, drink decaffeinated.

If you need that evening cup, or else you wake up with a headache, then you're not just chemically addicted, you're messing with a biochemical Pandora's Box that will lead you, later in life, to a daily fist full of pills to regulate cholesterol, blood pressure, and numerous forms of bowel and hormone dysfunctions. And you dick will die young, too.

Keep daily consumption of caffeinated drinks to a cup or two, preferably early in the day.

Let's Talk Liver

When your auto mechanic says you'll get better gas mileage if your fuel injectors were clean, you understand that. Poor gas mileage is the only way your car can exhibit this kind of ED—engine dysfunction. You can still get out on the road, even drive cross country if you wished, but the machine would perform much more efficiently if it was clean and well-tuned. This analogy works best for those of you who can get an erection, but can't hold it all the way to the finish line. You run out of gas too soon because of bad mileage.

Your body is the same, and not just with regard to ED. Most people think that all their internal organs are *healthy*, right up to the point that they are struck by disease.

Remember the guy that had never been sick a day in his life until suddenly, from out of nowhere, he was carted off to the hospital? It's not just about cancer; it applies to liver disease and the failure of other organs, too. Short of the onset of disease, your organs can perform sub-optimally, just like your fuel injectors. This is another case of sub-clinical dysfunction, and your liver, as a workhorse of bodily metabolism, is subject to overuse and abuse.

Your liver cleanses your body of many toxins by breaking them down, combining them with bile and letting you crap them away. It also metabolizes carbohydrates, proteins, and fat. It breaks down fat to produce energy, and it converts excess carbohydrates to fatty acids and triglycerides which are stored away in adipose tissue—body fat.

Your liver is a metabolic machine. It has a maximum capacity. Like the old Lucille Ball routine, when too much raw product comes along the conveyor belt, things get fouled up.

When your liver is called upon to do too many things, such as neutralizing all the artificial flavorings, dyes, partially hydrogenated oils, and process extraordinary amounts of alcohol and fat all at once, it is depleted of the enzymes it needs to perform its job. Things don't shut down completely—when they do, you wind up in the hospital—but poor digestion, disease, and malaise will ensue.

It will critically affect your ability to produce an erection.

Chapter 16: Your Prostate

A vibrant prostate gland is essential for maintaining health and extending your sex life. It is also a fundamental part of the pleasure you experience at the crucial moment.

First, what is the prostate? The prostate is a gland that wraps around your urethra, the tube that carries urine from your bladder to your penis. It provides most of the seminal fluid when you ejaculate. Sperm are added via a duct from your *vas deferens* and seminal vesicles, storage tanks for sperm which produce additional fluid necessary for ejaculation.

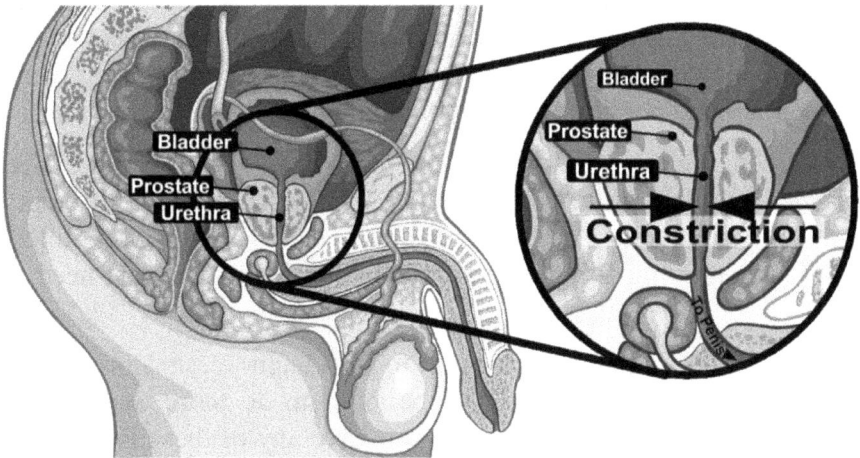

Did you know that the cartilage in your nose never stops growing? An analogous effect is operating on your prostate. Most men who are in their fifties experience some enlargement of their prostate gland which becomes more pronounced as the decades roll by.

Recent advancements in understanding how to stay healthy have allowed us to be feisty, fun-loving, and fully functional until we are past our sixties, and I'd like to think that this book will permit you to join in the party on your eightieth birthday, celebrating with a *Bang!*

But unhealthy living allows—in fact, encourages—the growth of your prostate to continue until it becomes a problem.

Your urethra is the tube that carries urine from your bladder to the outside world. Your prostate gland *surrounds* your urethra. As your prostate enlarges, it presses and constricts the urethra. Many men suffer from excessive prostate growth resulting in their urethra being all but pinched off. It's like stepping on a garden hose.

BPH—benign prostatic hyperplasia—is the condition of having your prostate grow too large—hyperplasia. It is benign in that the growth itself if not threatening; benign means NOT malignant. If the architecture was such that the urethra was outside the prostate, BPH would probably never be of note outside of medical academia.

But we do notice. Symptoms of BPH include the need to pee often, the need to go frequently during the night, difficulty beginning to pee, a slow stream that stops and starts and then stops again while peeing, and the possibility of dribbling after having peed.

When the constriction of the urethra is so obstructive that bladder muscles can't push urine past the "pinch," you can't empty yourself. Your bladder remains half—or more—filled. Consequently, you fill up again quickly and have an urgent need to pee.

BIG NOTE: Before you begin to self-diagnose, understand that these symptoms, may be a sign of more serious conditions, perhaps cancer. If you have any of these issues, see your doctor, now!

The *cavernous nerves* which are essential for you to get an erection run across the surface of the prostate gland and adhere to it. Removing them from the prostate has been described by surgeon Dr. Patrick Walsh as "peeling a wet tissue, undamaged, from a surface." Still, if prostate cancer is detected early enough, the possibility of saving these nerves is increased; you can still function sexually without a prostate, but not without these nerves.

In short, let your doctor stick his finger in your butt for a few moments and check you out. Not only won't it kill you, it may save your life and Harry's.

Also, get a PSA test. Prostate Specific Antigen can be measured in a blood test. The level of PSA in your blood can help detect cancer of the prostate early. Additionally, recent studies indicate—not absolutely conclusively—that establishing a baseline PSA level in one's forties may predict the likelihood or unlikelihood of prostate cancer in one's sixties. Forewarned is forearmed.

This begs the question, what can we do to ensure a long lived and happy prostate gland? Surprise, I've already told you:

• Eat healthy fruits and vegetables. Include fish in your diet. Avoid excessively fatty foods.

• Exercise frequently. Get out there for thirty minutes every few days and work up to three, four, or five days a week of thirty to sixty minutes of sweat. Sex does not count toward this time!

• Go easy—at least, easier—on the booze. Enjoy beer, wine and hard liquor responsibly, not just with regard to driving, but also with regard to the assault on your body.

• Spank the monkey with some regularity. By spank the monkey, of course, I mean stretch the bungee. You know, polish the putter, shampoo Kojak, plunk the magic twanger, Froggie (gotta be over fifty to understand that one). Pet your sperm whale. Finally, if you like Star Wars allusions: test fire the death star, tickle Yoda behind the ears, or Hand Solo.

Dr. Graham Giles of The Cancer Council Victoria in Melbourne, Australia, observed, based on research he concluded in 2003, that frequent ejaculation is key to a healthy prostate later in life. The implication is that frequency should occur earlier in life. Men who ejaculate four or five times per week while in their twenties, regardless of the methodology used, have a lower incidence of prostate disorder or disease later in life. He states that increased frequency of ejaculation up to age fifty is a predictor of reduced issues later on.

This information, which could easily have been labeled an urban legend, has actually been around for quite a while, though the evidence had been entirely anecdotal.

An under- or un-exercised prostate accumulates toxins the same as blood and lymph. Ejaculation blows out the sludge.

Preferred frequency is three to four times per week. That doesn't mean that if you're getting great sex two or three times you should feel compelled to slap another one off just to round up your averages; if it truly is "great" sex, you probably will be disinclined to do so, anyway.

Great sex—the kind that gets you turbo aroused—results in a deeper and fuller orgasm and ejaculation. Greater arousal causes you to come from a deeper place within your testes, and ejaculate younger and more vital sperm. You clean the pipes more effectively.

However, if you're only fortunate enough to have your lady's attention once per week, or less often, forget childhood parental admonitions or damnation from the pulpit... choke the bishop at long stoplights if you have to.

Chapter 17: Vitamins and Nutritional Supplements

It's best to get your vitamins and minerals in whole, natural foods that are rich in essential nutrients, rather than get them in pills, capsules, or potions. With that understanding, supplements are useful when you are unsure as to whether you are getting everything you need to leverage your health goals through nutrition.

Supplements are supplied as pills, capsules, and some liquid preparations that deliver a wide spectrum of nutritionally important compounds, vitamins, and minerals. If you're missing something from your food, supplements—as the name clearly states—*top you off* with what you haven't gotten in your regular diet. They are convenient and confer health benefits.

However, taking supplements as your primary source of nutrition is not reliable:

- Science does not have a comprehensive list of *everything* a body needs. In the 1990s a class of compounds, *phytonutrients*, were discovered. They include over 10,000 separate chemicals that confer essential health to humans which, before this time, nutritional science didn't even know existed.
- Therefore, there are no supplements which contain these substances as they are still largely unclassified, unidentified, and unable to be synthesized; it just isn't possible to prepare a pill with everything you can get in a grape, leaf of spinach, or an apple. There are no supplements or combination of supplements that contain everything you need to be healthy.
- Many of the most important nutritional elements must be supplied to your body in their natural context to be effective. Removed, purified, or synthesized, they just don't work as they do in nature.

So, on the one hand, nobody knows everything your body needs, and on the other, even if we did, preparing a pill with all those compounds just isn't possible, and if we could, they still wouldn't be as effective as getting the nutrient in food.

We Don't Know What We Don't Know

Because we don't have a comprehensive knowledge of all the health-compounds in natural foods, preparing a vitamin in the laboratory, or extracting a nutrient from a fruit takes it out of context. Nature didn't know that a pharmaceutical company was going to imitate it and make a compound in the lab. Nature didn't know it was supposed to tell pharmacologists, "Oh, don't forget to add some X, Y, and Z to that vitamin pill otherwise it won't work as well."

So companies churn out every vitamin in its own bottle, and every cofactor in its own box, but without the subtle harmony of a natural mixture, much of it is just peed or pooped away. When a vitamin is eaten as food, it is absorbed faster, in higher concentrations, and is more effective at doing what it's supposed to do. Those substances benefit us and encourage Harry. So, the green leafy vegetable is better than the supplement, but supplements are still important because we live in a real world and we don't always eat as properly as we should.

Not All Supplements are Created Equal

This section, with regard to the quality of supplements, is excerpted from Dr. Alison Brooks' *How We Can Stop Promoting Autism in Our Children*:

> Pretty packaging and high price tags do not ensure a quality product. In my practice, I personally use supplements that come from a company I have worked with for more than 20 years. This company has its own FDA approved lab … and has a drug license. Every batch of raw material, regardless of where it comes from, even with long term trusted sources, is tested. And if it doesn't meet their criteria it is rejected.
>
> This lab tests each supplement as it is being manufactured. The finished product is then tested once again for potency. This company also ensures full potency of ALL ingredients up to the

expiration date. One can entirely trust that what appears on the label is actually in the product.

This just isn't so for many brands—including the most popular advertised brands one sees on store shelves.

While everyone loves a bargain, there are some problems with shopping for supplements using only price as a guide. The following are five good questions you should ask buying *any* supplement:

1. Does the company actually make the vitamin? Many companies do not. They merely place their labels on the product and market them. The labeling company will do no quality control on these products.

2. Are the ingredients listed on the label contained in the product? Often times, they are not, or not in the concentrations stated on the label. Most companies rely on a Certificate of Assay. This document is provided by the seller of the product to the labeling company. However, most don't test to confirm the assay. There are no rules governing these practices. No records are required, and no one is accountable. *Caveat emptor.*

3. Are the products tested for quality or for contaminants? It's best to find a company that makes its products, and tests for quality and purity. You should know where the materials came from. Most of the botanicals purchased in America come from the Far East and require scrutiny before they are distributed.

4. How is the tablet or capsule made? Something as simple as how a tablet is produced can affect the *bioavailability*. Many manufacturers use inert ingredients that interfere with the absorption of the nutrients. Capsules generally have less inert material than tablets. In general, capsules are better absorbed than supplements in tablets, but even capsules may contain inert ingredients that interfere with absorption.

5. How long will the supplement keep its potency on the shelf? This is another "label claims" issue. Vitamins break down over time. Will the label be accurate after six months? A year? Is there a clear expiration date on the vitamins? A good company

will put more of each ingredient into the capsule or tablet so that the label claims will be true through the expiration date.

I've provided a link to Dr. Brooks' web site, NatOpt.com, in the final section of this book. She offers a line of high quality supplements that conform to these essential parameters. Buy them where you wish, but this should provide you with a base-line.

Nitric Oxide—Part III

So what supplements do you take to pump up the nitric oxide? Here are a few suggestions that will support your body's natural nitric oxide production. But by themselves, they may not work; enjoy them only in the context of a healthier lifestyle.

- Folic acid

- L-arginine

- Propionyl-L-carnitine.

- Zinc: If your diet doesn't keep your levels of zinc as high as it should, then a multivitamin with minerals is suggested

- Gingko: there's no positive proof, but in studies of men who were taking anti-depressants—discussed earlier as Harry-killers—the anti-erectile effect of these drugs was lessened.

- Saw-Palmetto, an herb

- Anti-oxidants (very important) including vitamins A, C, D, E

- Omega-3 fish oil, specifically DHA.

You'll see other supplements mentioned in the literature, but if you spend more time eating healthier organic foods, and cutting down—or out—those things you currently eat that are killing Harry, you don't have to empty your wallet on supplements.

Chapter 18: Things That Harm Harry

Allergies

An allergy can begin at any time in life. You may be fine with Fluffy the cat for years and then you start reacting to its fur and dander. Allergists and medical researchers don't know why the immune system suddenly decides it doesn't like some substance to which you have had no previous sensitivity, but you can be eighty-years-old and develop an entirely new allergy.

Just to clarify, an allergy is an immune response. The body's reaction to invading bacteria—for example—is good. It kills the bacteria and maintains health. When the body responds to a substance in the environment that poses no threat, we call it an allergy. The substance that elicits the response is labeled an allergen. An allergic reaction can range from a mild irritation of the skin or membranes (nose, eye, lungs, etc.) to anaphylactic shock that can be deadly.

A major proportion of the population of the United States has become allergic to gluten, the ubiquitous protein in wheat discussed earlier. One symptom of food-allergies is fatigue, especially an hour or two after a meal. Some research has shown a link between gluten, specifically, and the tiredness that is often associated with hitting the 3:00PM wall. It's just one more factor in your overall toxic load.

The Sign of the Beast is [TV]

If there ever was one single detriment to the health of Americanized people—those that subscribe to western dietary extravagances—it is television. Not just that it's a passive, sit-on-your-ass activity, but television viewing—in the United States—puts you in the line of fire of the onslaught of commercials that are designed to get you to eat the worst possible poisons even when you're not hungry.

The purveyors of these messages don't even care if you buy the product they're promoting, as long as you go to your kitchen and eat. They act as a pack. They inundate the airwaves with messages designed to elicit a craving.

Perhaps you go for the frozen pizza. The next it's chips. The chip advertiser doesn't care if you're heating up the frozen pizza because when the pizza commercial comes, the pizza is already gone and you'll go for the chips.

It's a conspiracy to deprive you of sex. *Those bastards!*

Round and round. They advertise, you eat, then you then restock from the supermarket, and again you subject yourself to their mind-numbing messages. It never ends.

This is psychological terrorism of the kind that will get you fat, piss away your money on crap food, and ruin your dick.

Erectile health—all health—demands the management of recreational or sport eating: that which is not associated with hunger.

Junk food, the kind hyped in the majority of TV commercials, is high in unsaturated fat, high fructose corn syrup, gluten, and a cadre of chemical preservatives, stabilizers and colorings that you can't pronounce and your body can't tolerate. These are the worst offenders and they add to your toxic load.

They kill Harry!

Eating Just Before Sleep

You watch TV before bedtime, and perhaps while in bed. You eat. If you choose to embark on a healthy lifestyle or one healthy enough to rid you of erectile dysfunction, this is counterproductive. Eating at this time loads you with empty calories and bowel-poisoning chemicals.

Excess calories have no choice but to be converted to fat, and chemicals linger in your circulatory and lymphatic system longer than they might otherwise, as you remain motionless in bed for hours after they hit your system.

Exotic Fruit and Berry "Miracle" Supplements

At one time or another, you have seen an infomercial, heard or news blurb, been invited to a living room presentation, or sat in a Starbucks while some wannabe Multi-Level-Marketing superstar beat you up about some exotic fruit or berry drink, powder, or pill that gives you the same energy as eight solid hours of sleep, wipes out cancer, and improves the resale value of your automobile.

First, these products are a poor Band-Aid. Even if they actually could do what they are purported to do, they're just covering up the result of your terrible food, drink, and lifestyle choices.

Second, the pharmacologically effective dose of the active ingredient—the amount you'd have to actually consume for the product to do what it says it does if it could do it—is so high that you'd drown trying to down enough to de-flame you. This is true for the most prominently advertised supplements, including those that provide the active ingredient in red wine: resveratrol. To get benefit, you'd have to take a prohibitively expensive quantity, popping pills several times a day. Same for acai berry.

Not to be too much of a cynic, but if the active ingredients of these preparations worked, big Pharm would have figured out some way to patent it, and then mark it up a million percent at the retail counter.

The road to good health for a long, healthy life, along with effective rejuvenation of Harry, is to moderate, or completely avoid the terrible food, drink, and lifestyle choices as described throughout this book.

The reason I included this discussion of miracle drinks and powders in the "Harmful" category, is because the average human psyche is such that if you believe you are doing something that is positive and healthy, you may take certain latitudes at other times.

You will negotiate with yourself. "I had my miracle berry earlier, so I can have an extra portion of char-grilled, grease-laden ribs now."

I don't delude myself into thinking you're not going to have the ribs anyway. But any negotiation must be an honest one. Eat the ribs, but find something substantial to give in return: work out an extra day that week, skip dessert, or don't drink for three days. The berry drink doesn't count.

Pain Killers & Anti-Depressants

Read the warnings on your bottle of acetaminophen and ibuprofen. These non-prescription, over the counter pain killers are murder on your liver. Reminder: your liver is the major organ of detoxification that rids your body of inflammation causing compounds; overtax your liver and your dick dies.

The evidence suggests that these drugs, when taken in the recommended dose, do no harm. However, exceed the recommended dose and liver failure can ensue. Another reminder: your liver won't fail by turning off, it will slow down, work inefficiently, and cause disease in other parts of the body.

Many prescription, non-prescription, and recreational drugs kill libido. This will diminish your ability to achieve erection. Anti-depressants, such as Prozac®, Zoloft® and others include in their warnings that they may have "sexual side effects." Sexual side effects in men = Erectile Dysfunction. And it's not "may," it's *will*.

Only if you stop taking them might you retrieve your potency; do this only under the supervision of your doctor, but seek that supervision right away.

Author's note: perhaps if you got laid from time to time you wouldn't be so damned depressed!

An Important Note for Bicycle Riders

This discussion is about physical damage to the nerves and blood vessels that control the erectile mechanism.

Whether you're an enthusiast that spends hours each week spinning over hill and dale, or just a casual weekend rider, beware the damage you could do to yourself due to a poorly positioned or badly fitting bicycle seat.

Your *perineum* is that area between your anus and scrotum (vagina in women). Through that thin area run the dorsal artery of the penis, the deep artery of the penis and the dorsal nerve of the penis. For women, the dorsal nerve of the clitoris replaces its male analog, so advise your ladies of this issue as well.

These blood vessels and nerves can be compressed and damaged when they are squeezed between the bicycle seat and the *pubic arch* of your pelvis. As an avid rider in my younger days, I remember my dick going numb while riding; there were fewer options then.

I'm riding again; it's my primary exercise. The first time I got back on the saddle, however, I could feel that uncomfortable pressure between my legs. But now, I had the savvy to go directly to the local bike shop, describe my discomfort and—*voila*—I had a comfortable seat installed and I was out the door.

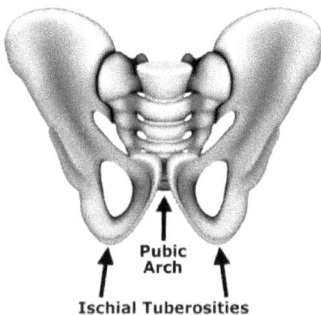

Pubic Arch

Ischial Tuberosities

The key is to use a seat that properly supports you on your *Ischial Tuberosities*—the two protruding parts of your pelvis. When cycling, you don't sit on your butt cheeks as you do in a lounge chair. On a bicycle, your body is supported at these bones. A poorly fitting seat that is too narrow or positioned badly will slip you forward so the saddle slides up between your legs into the pubic arch; this puts pressure on the arteries and nerves that go directly to Harry crushing the vessels and nerves that go to your pecker under the entire weight of your body. Got it Lance?

Prolonged abuse can cause permanent damage to the arteries, nerves, or both. This is the kind of erectile dysfunction that you really don't want to have—physical injury to the apparatus.

Unfit for Fitness?

I discussed the importance of the Psoas Stretch to relieve pressure on your lower back and reduce irritation of the nerves that control erection. This will also improve lower back elasticity and reduce pain in this region of your body for use both in and out of bed.

I also described air cycling, the exercise designed to improve lymphatic drainage from your lower body, thereby assisting in cleansing toxins from Chez Harry.

Now we have to take it one step further. Are you too unfit for sex? When you have that erection and are about to satisfy your woman, will the rest of your body perform well enough to go the distance?

Body pain will kill a hard-on, even while you're having sex, as quickly as hearing a male voice call "Hi honey, I'm home," coming from the downstairs foyer.

If your stomach or leg muscles are cramping, or your lungs are burning, you're increasing your chances—given your history of ED—of losing an erection that shouldn't be lost, and at the worst possible moment.

Sexual stamina is not a term that refers specifically to your erection. Muscular endurance and lung capacity are necessary to keep the rhythm, maintain the demanded force of penetration, and to allow you to vary your motion—enhance her satisfaction—to the very end. If you're a considerate lover, you'll want to keep going a little longer, past your ejaculation, just in case she has one more bullet still in the chamber. If you're not sure, then ASK!

Remember, there is no "I" in ORGASM. Then again, there's no "P" either, but every once and a while a woman may let go with a squirt. (It's not really pee, but the joke doesn't work the other way.)

You can follow all the directives in this book, and get Harry's full cooperation. This doesn't guarantee that you won't wind up being lousy in bed. So, while I'm not going to discuss technique, I am going to remind you that you need to have some lung capacity and body strength to properly make love to your lady. Further, if you want to vary position and sexual style, you most likely will need some upper body power as well.

As they say on all the advertisements for ED meds, "...check with your doctor to make sure you're healthy enough for sexual activity."

An essential difference between popping boner pills and following the suggestions in this book is that the ED medications do nothing to help you be fit enough for sex, while following these recommendations as part of a daily routine, most certainly will.

And finally: Briefs vs. Boxers

The perennial issue. Heat reduces the production of testosterone in the testes. Some mammalian species keep their balls inside until they are needed; then they descend, externalize, cool down, and pump up the action. After rutting season, they retract so they won't get caught as the animal runs through the brush and brambles... ouch... and it dampens the sex urge in males outside mating season.

Nature put our jewels outside our human bodies. We have no rutting season. Our balls are in play all the time. But some jag-off thought that we needed clothes, so now we all run around dressed, even in warm weather. Boxers are slightly better for male performance. Briefs are better support during exercise and sports.

Wear what's comfortable.

Chapter 19: Weight Control and Weight Loss

We've come a long way. Several times I've stated that the recommendations in this book address overall health, not just erectile function. So I'd be remiss if I didn't address this issue.

The best weight loss is SLOW weight loss. Any diet that promises you will lose ten pounds in the first two weeks is pulling your chain. You can't do it, you can't sustain it, and you can't achieve healthy weight modification in this short amount of time.

There is a prevailing delusion that it's all about calories: just cut down on calorie intake, and increase exercise to burn off calories, and the scale will swing in your favor.

Unfortunately, once you've crossed into your forties, that won't work anymore. The biochemistry changes, the dynamics of fat production and storage change, and the requirements for burning fat shift. It's all different.

If you're not sure if you're fat, look for the jiggle on your belly and what hangs from your arms and neck. The arc your belly takes when it leaves your chest and extends outward before returning to your pecker is good evidence. Can you still see your pecker?

And when you're losing weight, you don't need a scale. Measure your progress by the fit of your clothes. Pick out a snug pair of jeans and always compare how they feel when you put them on after they have just been washed. Clean jeans are snugger than those that have been worn a few times. It's that first wearing that shows you how you're doing.

The Three Keys to Mature Weight Loss

The rules are different when you pass into your forties, and get more difficult as the decades roll by. It's not just about cutting down on calories, portion control, and exercise. Not anymore. Because all calories are not the same.

Merely cutting down on calories puts your body into starvation metabolism. Rather than go to fat for energy, your system will begin to break down protein—muscle. Men past forty lose upper-body muscle-mass naturally. Trying to get rid of that gut can accelerate that process if you don't take into account the difference in calories consumed from different sources.

First, the three keys:

- We all eat too much, so *Portion Control* is important. Taking in fewer chemicals, less gluten, fewer inflammants, along with fewer calories to slow weight gain is an easy first step.

- Exercise: any weight control or weight loss program that does not include a combination of aerobic and light upper body weight training just won't work. It's the addition of muscle-building that must be added when past forty.

- *Increase the inclusion of foods that have a low Glycemic index* in your diet, with the reduction of those with a high index. While this is important for everyone from children on up, it is the critical component of weight loss in later years.

> *The Glycemic Index* is a measure of how quickly a food causes a rise in blood sugar. High glycemic foods cause a rapid rise with a spike in insulin production. These are the foods which promote weight gain and poor health. The index runs zero to one-hundred; one-hundred being equal to the effect of eating pure glucose.

Let's discuss the nature of getting fat, and then come back to the three keys.

I could include a comprehensive chart of common foods and their Glycemic Index ratings. I won't. There are dozens available— free on the web. *Items with a glycemic index above 50 should be avoided, while Items with an index 50 or below are to be embraced.* Unfortunately, the highest rated on most charts is beer.

Take a look at any of the charts. Run your eyes down the listing and what you see will be obvious:

- HIGH Glycemic foods. Index above 50: White flour products (breads); all sweet and sugary snacks including things with honey; greasy and fried foods (French fries, potato chips); starchy foods including starchy vegetables (potatoes, carrots, corn, rice); pasta; pumpkin, watermelon, raisons

- MARGINAL Glycemic foods, Index around 50: Whole wheat or bran bread; basmati rice; sweet potatoes; whole wheat pasta

- LOW Glycemic foods. Index below 50: Whole grain pasta; pumpernickel bread; oatmeal; wild rice; fresh fruit; soy and peanuts (raw, not in oil); green vegetables have an index below 15.

Weight loss occurs when you reduce your Glycemic Load, which is determined by:

- The cumulative average of the Glycemic Index of all the foods you eat.

- The quantity of those foods.

- The quantity of carbohydrates you eat as part of those foods.

Yeah, you knew we were going to get back to carbs at some point. But it's not only about the carbs. Reduce the carbohydrate laden foods at each meal by replacing them with vegetables, and other green stuff. Do not snack carb-heavy. And don't carbo-load unless you're a marathon runner. Jogging under nine miles (15K) will barely get all the glycogen (circulating calories in your blood and tissues) out of your system, so your Sunday run is not an alibi to load-up on Saturday night.

Why We Tend to Get Fat

Long ago, when our ancestors were still hunter-gatherers seeking food, and downing the occasional antelope or wildebeest, everything was wonderful. Everyone prospered and families grew and there was plenty for everyone. None of them looked like Daryl Hannah.

Then drought hit. Drought causes famine. Food was harder to find. Stress grew—eustress—good stress—as these early humans fought the elements to survive.

Everyone went into starvation, but within the population, a few of these early people had an unusual metabolism, a very tiny difference, not for any reason at all, just a genetic aberration, a part of the normal diversity of the human species. But this unusual genetic feature caused a few to burn less fat when under the stress of reduced calorie intake, i.e., less food.

It dropped their internal metabolic rate; their genetic makeup shut down nonessential functions of their bodies. They burned fewer calories, preserving what they had stored in their body fat.

Each individual was forced to live on what they had stored within themselves. It was something they couldn't share. Those whose bodies naturally burned calories at a *higher* rate, consumed their body fat more quickly. Many died. But a sufficient number of those whose metabolism slowed under the stress of the famine, survived until food was again available. They—the survivors—passed on that tiny extra metabolic advantage to their offspring; over generations, it became predominant genetic makeup of the tribe.

The next time there was a drought and subsequent famine, more people survived. However, if the next famine lasted longer, those people whose bodies were *slightly better still* at slowing metabolism survived the longer famine while others could not. These survivors, again, were able to pass that advantage onto their children... and round and round for thousands of generations and famines.

And now you've got it. You've got the gene that slows down your metabolism when food is scarce. Nature, however, is not perfect, and sometimes it over-shoots its mark.

If you just don't get around to eating, or think you'll skip a meal—breakfast or lunch—to "save" those calories for dinner, your body quickly begins to think FAMINE! Within hours a slight decrease in metabolic rate is measurable. You're burning fewer calories even though you're performing the same activities. You're not saving calories for dinner; you're accumulating calorie debt.

You may have heard that breakfast is the most important meal of the day. If for no other reason, this statement is true because that early meal primes your metabolism to burn calories at a higher rate, keeping the fire going.

Fasting

There is evidence that an occasional full-day fast, taking in nothing other than pure, clean water, confers health. It gives your body a day with no toxic load.

While one's metabolic rate slows, obviously it doesn't stop. Calories are burned and a small amount of stored fat is put into play.

Bowels empty. Without food, your liver rests. Toxins are pumped, being peed and pooped away.

Try it once a month. Twice if you can.

Fat-O-Stat versus Rapid Weight Loss

Just as a thermostat regulates the heating and air conditioning in your home to maintain a constant temperature, you have a metabolic fat-o-stat that maintains a constant amount of fat on your body. There is a genetic component to the fat-o-stat, but fortunately, like the thermostat, it can be adjusted.

The fat-o-stat can be raised or lowered by slow changes in the amount of fat on your body. Operative word: "Slow."

Ever really pigged-out for a weekend and were sure that you must have gained five pounds? Were you surprised when you didn't? The fat-o-stat resisted a sudden gain in weight, passing off excess calories. This isn't healthy. It screws with your blood triglyceride levels and all sort of other bodily functions. So, don't test this every weekend.

If you've ever pigged-out for an entire week on a vacation, or gluttonized for weeks during the Holidays, you may have been certain you gained five pounds. Were you surprised when you got to a scale and realized you gained *ten?*

You can easily overrun the fat-o-stat and, in the process, reset it to a higher level.

On the flipside, did you ever go on a "20 pounds in 20 days" diet, do great, buy pants a waist size smaller and then have them be too tight to wear within a month's time? Your fat-o-stat again; it adjusted your metabolism to increase your bodily fat ratio back up to where it was set.

The fat-o-stat attempts to keep your body fat constant. It's the metabolic feedback mechanism responsible for survival during famine as discussed previously.

Unfortunately for modern men and women, it is much easier to adjust the fat-o-stat UP than down. There is no natural pressure for downward adjustment: "Hey body, there's too much food, let's get skinny." That just doesn't happen.

You may want to take a deep breath before reading further, but... and this isn't a joke... *people used to stop eating when they were full.*

Early man was rarely overweight as survival required a physical lifestyle. They ate when they could and what they could. There were no nacho chips or chocolate covered peanuts to eat on impulse.

A note for anthropologists: I acknowledge that there are some populations among whom storage of large amounts of body fat had a cultural and evolutionary advantage. To this day, men and women of these peoples may be very large by Western standards; you're just not one of them.

The key to adjusting the fat-o-stat downward is to do it slowly. About one pound per week stays below the fat-o-stat's radar. That's just over two ounces a day. It won't even show up on your scale, yet it amounts to fifty pounds per year. Wow.

Unless you're 6'6" tall, if you're fifty pounds overweight, you're "morbidly obese." That's a technical term based on a Body Mass Index (BMI). BMI was never meant to be used to assess individuals. Its creator measured populations of people. Applying BMI to individuals is bogus and should be ignored. Its adoption into the lexicon of nutritionists demonstrates how out of touch that profession is.

Still, morbid obesity generally means that your excess fat will impact your health. *And you're reading this book because of one of those affects*. The next affect may be the onset of diabetes or a heart attack.

The majority of fat people will benefit greatly by losing fifty, forty, or even twenty pounds (9 kg.) to start. Think of three or six months—a year is better—as the time period in which to set your goal. Modest loss, slow but consistent, is doable. It took you ten years to put it on, consider yourself lucky you can lose it in just one.

The carrot: it will likely revive Harry, as well as make you more attractive so that someone will *want* to have sex with you.

The fat-o-stat will get accustomed to the lower fat content of your body and adjust itself down; it does not resist these slow movements in body weight. It does, however, lag behind weight loss. You must lower your body weight and keep in there before the fat-o-stat resets itself to a slimmer you.

And here's where the scale is not your friend. Because the weight loss regimen I suggest includes muscle building, your weight might increase a bit before it drops because muscle is much heavier than fat. A small increase in muscle affects the scale a lot more than a drop of an inch at the waist.

> ***Special Note:*** It is unhealthy in the long run to yo-yo diet. Lose weight, then gain weight, then lose it again, then gain it all back, plus an extra pound or two. Very unhealthy. It stresses your organs, wreaks havoc on

your endocrine system and, ultimately, messes with Harry.

Exercise

How about walking a mile a day? A calm walking pace is three miles per hour; one mile in twenty minutes. Some cardiovascular benefit is achieved if you get that down to a fifteen to seventeen-minute mile. If you can jog it in ten minutes, you'll feel great, but work up to that slowly. Consult your physician.

A ten-minute mile—six mph—is doable for almost anyone, but you may have to work up to it over a period of months.

Remember that gym membership you've been paying on for the past fourteen years? Do the math. You've probably spent close to $750 per hour for the time you've actually been there.

Getting back into the regimen of working-out is not an all-or-nothing affair. You don't have to get into upper body and aerobic exercise all at the same time. Your immediate need is to get your body moving. That's what you need for sex.

If you get winded walking a flight of stairs or running down to the end of the driveway to get the paper, then you just can't have good sex. How often do you expect to be invited back after she goes through the experience of having you flop around on her gasping for air like a beached whale?

Regardless of your age, if the rest of your body fails to be a reliable delivery mechanism for Harry, then it's all for naught.

You must get your heart rate and breathing to the point where you're working up a reasonable sweat and you must keep it there for at least thirty minutes at a time. Sixty, if you're really serious about it.

After you've worked you way up to it, the first twenty minutes of any exercise session is solely preparing your body to begin cardio enhancement or fat-burn. If you only do twenty minutes, there will be little or no benefit.

When you do thirty minutes, you're really only getting a ten minute workout. Unless you're training for a particular athletic event, much more than an hour doesn't provide return with regard to rejuvenating Harry, or overall benefit for the non-athlete. That's why about sixty minutes is optimal.

You must get upper body exercise to offset your body's attempt to grab protein from your chest, back and arm muscles. Use a machine or free weights. Make sure you're feeling the exertion and—in the beginning—you should feel sore from stressing those myofibrils; that's what mobilizes the body to build more muscle. B*uild up slowly.* Do what you can without hurting yourself. Being bedridden with body pain is not going to help you get in shape. Consult your physician before beginning a fitness regimen. Buy a few lessons from a trainer to make sure you're using the equipment properly.

Chest, back, shoulders and arms. Work them to gain definition—even at your age—and to improve your weight loss regimen. The calories you burn will be from fat, not your muscle.

> ***Yet another warning:*** You will have gotten your full physical exam before beginning your exercise program. You'll understand your limitations based on your back, neck, and joint issues, and perhaps seek a professional trainer—at the gym or elsewhere—to advise you on how to accomplish your goals without doing yourself harm.

Chapter 20: The Punch Line

Everything I'm telling you affects your main man. Erectile dysfunction IS the effect of the stress you put on your body by eating the wrong things, combining food improperly, poisoning yourself both chemically and psychologically, and by sitting around like a fucking slug.

Yo-yo and fad dieting, pills and energy drinks that mess with your metabolism, and other extraordinary measures, all performed honorably enough with the aim of getting back into shape may be doing exactly the opposite. They take a toll on your body.

If you're not a lifelong athlete, you will not become one in your fifties. Sure, there's a magazine article about some guy that did it, but there's also a news story about the guy that got shot through his brain with a nail gun and survived... wanna try that, too?

Let's deal with realistic goals and strive toward achievable outcomes. You want your dick to work and perform reliably. You don't have to be an athlete, you don't have to be ripped, you don't even have to be *in shape*, whatever that is.

You just have to be fit enough for your blood vessels to pump up and maintain the pressure in your pecker. You need to be sure the neural messages moving up and down your spinal cord get to where they have to go. You also have to be able to go the distance without your heart exploding and your lungs collapsing. For that, you have to be, not perfectly, but sufficiently fit.

Of course it wouldn't hurt if you were attractive—remember, that's in the eye of the beholder—for your current woman, or some future prospect to invite you to her bed.

All the advice I've given you about eating organic and properly balanced foods, and drinking pure, clean water, are directed at the load on your liver. Toxins accumulate in your blood and your tissues because the liver just can't get rid of them all. Fat accumulates on and in your body because proper fat metabolism suffers under the strain of the volume of food and the poor quality of what you eat. Your liver just can't handle the load.

It is important to understand all the advice I've presented regarding stress, the metabolic impact on your adrenals and other endocrine glands, and the psychological overload to which we subject ourselves. These assault our bodies in ways that science does not yet fully understand. But the effect is there.

If you don't ever change the oil in your car, it will stop running, or run so poorly that every ride to the supermarket is an adventure. We abuse our bodies by neglect, failing to exercise in favor of choosing the easy, sedentary path each time we have that choice. It makes us physically less attractive and starts to shut down body functions. Your dick is one of them. Your ability to enjoy other fun activities is also impacted—in some cases, reduced to the point of extinction.

Your body doesn't understand that even though you're only in your fifties or sixties, you've got a lot of life to live. By your lifestyle you tell it otherwise, pouring toxins into your bloodstream and allowing them to fester.

If there's any chance that you can get an invitation to a fine woman's bed, you want to be "up and running." I think I've made a solid case for how you can do that. It worked for me and I intend to be sowing my oats well into my eighties... perhaps beyond.

So, along with long walks by the beach, and snuggling in front of the fire, and doing crosswords on Sunday morning, be sure that your Internet dating profile states quite clearly that you really enjoy sex, too.

PART IV: Immediate Action

Chapter 21: The One-Week Challenge

The Single Thing You Can Do to Restore Potency in 7 Days

You've read the book. Some suggestions make sense to you, and perhaps you'll try a few. Others don't, and you'll ignore those. But what if I told you that you could do one thing—and perhaps for as little as a week—that would bring Harry back enough to satisfy you and your partner.

You've likely heard of Celiac disease, an allergy to gluten in wheat and several other grains that results in severe intestinal pain and GI dysfunction.

"Gluten-Free" is now a badge of honor on food packaging, implying that the contents confer health. In a bass-ackwards way, it may be true. Not that they are healthy, but that they contribute less to making you sick.

A tsunami of recent research reveals that most people are affected by gluten, even if they exhibit none of the extreme symptoms of celiac. This reaction is detectable as a *systemic inflammation of blood vessels, nerves, and tissues of various organs.* Our old friend: sub-clinical inflammation.

More than any other single substance, gluten containing foods are present at almost every meal and in every snack. Could eliminating the inflammatory effects of gluten restore erectile function even if you do nothing else? I suspect that for some it may. There's only one way to find out if it will for you.

Avoid All Gluten for Seven Days.

That means no wheat, rye, barley, and a few other rarely used grains, but wheat is the heavy-hitter. Eliminating wheat means no bread or anything that looks like bread. No cereals, pastries, donuts, baked goods, or anything that doesn't conspicuously say, "Gluten-Free." Even ice cream often has gluten. Read labels carefully.

Rice and corn—including popcorn—are okay. Meat (all animal products), potatoes, eggs, cheese, vegetables, fruits, nuts, and seeds are all naturally gluten free.

It's the processed foods that you have to look out for. Even French fries, if they're not freshly made, may be dusted with wheat flour to keep them from sticking together in frozen preparations; they'll contain gluten

The rough part is resisting the urge to replace the satisfaction you get from breads and baked goods, by over-indulging in sugar and fried items. Do yourself a favor. Try not to use other foods as substitutes. *Eat meals. Avoid snacks. It's only seven days!*

Look for Benefits Above Your Belt, Too.

Everything in this book is about health, not just erectile health. The same strategies for restoring potency can get you off diabetes medications and *statins*, help you lose weight, clear brain-fog and lethargy, reduce joint pain and arthritis, avoid heart disease, reduce your risk of cancer, and more.

The One-Week Challenge is a single part of a larger puzzle for which there are many more pieces.

Whether this brings Harry back to life all by itself or not, it *will* improve your overall health. You'll sleep more soundly, wake rested, and not hit the 3:00PM wall. Overall, you'll feel better.

Your mood will elevate. Not only might your sexual performance improve, but your partner's interest in engaging you may also take a decided uptick, just because you won't be as much of an asshole.

Don't tell anyone what you're doing. Avoid gluten for seven solid days—no cheating—and don't be surprised when people comment about your looks and demeanor.

Remember: meat and potatoes are gluten free, but the bun on the hamburger is not. Be careful with ribs or anything with sauce because often they have gluten-containing thickeners and additives.

Eat meals. Avoid snacks. Try to work in a piece of fruit or small salad while you're at it. Use gluten-free dressings.

And if it works for you, consider going gluten-free for life. If it becomes part of your lifestyle, then the occasional transgression *won't* send you back to square one. Likely, you'll feel the difference when you have that bun or piece of cake, and you won't like what it does to you. You'll gladly choose not to do that again.

Don't let success undermine your long-term objective. If gluten-free is all you need to get an erection, that doesn't mean you shouldn't abide by some of the other health-giving practices discussed in the rest of this book so you'll live long, and Enjoy Healthy Sex for Life.

But note: Gluten is not the only offender. There are other foods, most notably processed and natural sugars that also inflame the body. So if gluten-free doesn't restore potency well enough—though it may give you more wood than you had before—that's what the rest of this book was about.

Let me know about your success via the publisher: Admin@HShirePublishing.com.

Acknowledgements

This book is primarily about Erectile Dysfunction. I worked on it mostly by myself, not wanting to advertise the fact that I had ED— past tense. Like Joey on *Friends* whose acting/modeling career put him on billboards for VD, I was afraid that no woman would give me a shot for fear of being disappointed. I got over that. And I got over the embarrassment factor as well.

However, I did enlist a few men to read the manuscript so I could get feedback about the "voice" of the writing, so they could let me know if any of the jokes worked. Out of respect for their privacy, and so as not to confuse their literary assistance with experiential contribution, I'm not going to mention their names.

I do thank them very much for their help, large and small, and will repay in man-currency... drinks are on me. Just one each. Form a line to the right. I will have to stamp your hand after you've redeemed your reward.

Sincerely, thanks to all.

Links and References

Please let us know if you hit any dead or incorrect links: Admin@HShirePublishing.com.

Robin's Blog for Men is an ongoing discussion of erectile dysfunction, and more importantly, **erectile function**, and other related topics: http://RobinsBlogForMen.blogspot.com

Quality Nutritional Supplements & Naturopathic counseling: http://www.NatOpt.com

IFOAM.org: International Federation of Organic Agricultural Movements. Source page for quotes in text:
http://www.ifoam.org/growing_organic/1_arguments_for_oa/food_q uality/f_quality_main_page.html

The Future of Food: About the movie, from their website:
> "*The Future of Food* offers an in-depth investigation into the disturbing truth behind the unlabeled, patented, genetically engineered foods that have quietly filled U.S. grocery store shelves for the past decade."

FineWaters.com: A resource for learning about available water providers, sources of water, and what constitutes pure, clean water.

Viagra® website: "Side effects:"
http://www.viagra.com/taking-viagra/viagra-side-effects.aspx

Cialis® website: "Safety:" http://www.cialis.com/Pages/safety.aspx

The Truth about Aspartame:
http://www.youtube.com/watch?v=lqIFDoOwSFM by Russell Blaylock, MD. See his credentials at:
http://www.russellblaylockmd.com/

Nightingale-Conant: *Lead the Field* by Earl Nightingale available at http://www.nightingale.com/LeadTheField

Some notes about butter:
http://www.drlwilson.com/articles/butter.htm

Robert Cohen: A warning about Milk:
http://www.youtube.com/watch?v=tYpafipJyDE and;

The *"Not Milk" website*: http://www.notmilk.com

Contact Robin via the publisher: Admin@HSHirePublishing.com

About the Author

Robin has a Master of Science degree in the biological sciences from Florida Atlantic University in Boca Raton, FL. Prior to moving to Florida he studied aerospace engineering at the Polytechnic Institute of Brooklyn, now part of the New York City University system.

Robin is also author of *Lose Weight with Nutritional Leverage: A Guide to Living Young as Long as Possible* available in print and e-Book from Amazon, Barnes & Noble, and others.

Robin says, "Nutritional Leverage is an eating and lifestyle regimen for total health and longevity. It sprung out of the research done for HARD! I just kept going. I lost a lot of weight, though that wasn't my initial purpose. But in deciding on a title, one just can't attract attention to a nutrition book without 'Lose Weight' in the title. So I pandered."

Currently living in Palm Beach County, Florida, Robin is an accomplished speaker and trainer, and is available to discuss his areas of expertise with groups and organizations.

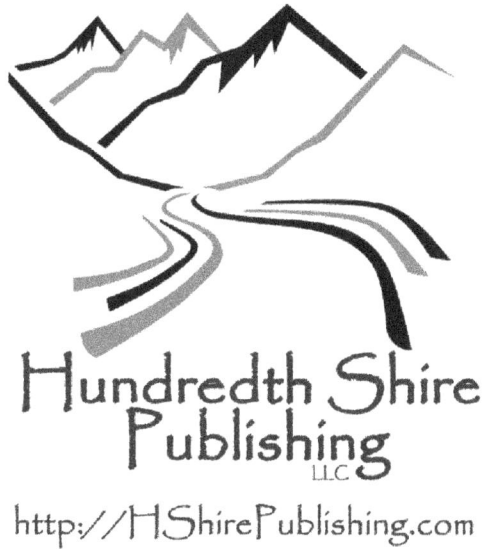

Hundredth Shire
Publishing
LLC
http://HShirePublishing.com

Other recent health publications include:

Lose Weight with Nutritional Leverage: a Guide to Living Young as Long as Possible, by Robin D. Ader, 2013

How We Can Stop Promoting Autism in Our Children: 2nd edition, by Dr. Alison Brooks, 2012

Available as print and eBook